Best - W<br>
John C

# YOU DON'T KNOW JOHN CAIN?

# YOU DON'T KNOW JOHN CAIN?

by
Pat Sykes
With an introduction by Alan Whittaker

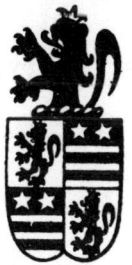

**VAN DUREN**
**GERRARDS CROSS 1979**

ISBN 0–905715–10–1

The photograph on the book jacket is by
David Marriott
All the illustrations in the book were supplied by
Mr. John Cain

Typeset by Inforum Ltd., Portsmouth
Printed and bound by A. Wheaton & Co. Ltd.,
Exeter, Devon

# Contents

# INTRODUCTION

## by

# ALAN WHITTAKER

"You don't know John Cain?" The taxi driver made no attempt to hide his incredulity as he threaded through the teeming traffic in the murk of a Merseyside dusk in mid-winter. I could see him surveying me with disbelief in the driving mirror as though I had arrived in Liverpool from a long sojourn in Outer Mongolia or Outer Space.

"I've heard of him, but I've never met him" I volunteered as we rattled towards the Mersey Tunnel and the road to Birkenhead where John Cain lives. "I've come from London to see him."

The driver digested this information and appeared pleased. "So they've heard of him down there in London have they? Everybody round here knows about him. He's a healer and I'm told he's very good. The best there is, so they reckon. What's the matter with you then? Back trouble? Most of 'em have back trouble, but he soon puts them right. People have gone to see him on crutches and come away walking like two-year olds. I've driven a lot of folk to see him and I'm told that sometimes they come in coaches. Imagine that, coach loads of people who have tried doctors and hospitals turning up on the doorstep of somebody who never went to medical school. It makes you think."

He drove on in silence, musing over the chain of thought the conversation had set in motion.

Since that first meeting with John Cain, just before Christmas in 1977, he has certainly given me plenty to think about. Hardly a week passes without his name cropping up as people from all parts of Britain – and countries all over the world – write to me or telephone asking for his address.

Let me explain. I've been a Fleet Street journalist for more than twenty years and in the winter of 1977 I decided to write a series of articles on unorthodox healers.

I mentioned this to a publisher friend and he said "Then you must see John Cain."

7

"And who is John Cain?" I asked. He told me enough to interest me and a few days later I caught a train to Liverpool and took a taxi from Lime Street Station to Cain's home. As a national newspaper reporter I have interviewed many healers. Some described themselves as Faith Healers, some as Spiritual Healers, others as Divine Healers. John Cain was different. "I don't know what I am" he smiled. "I just seem to be able to help people. I haven't given it a lot of thought but I suppose I must be some sort of channel. As long as it works that's all that matters, I'll let others try to figure it out."

It was typical of John Cain. Although he believes passionately that whatever gifts he possesses are from God, he does not cloak his work in mysticism or religious mumbo-jumbo.

Christians of all shades, Jews, Muslims, Buddhists and self-confessed agnostics have sought his help. He has also demonstrated his remarkable powers in Japan where he won glowing tributes from scientists.

A former blacksmith John Cain is as tough and uncompromising as the tools of his trade – the anvil, the glowing forge and raw metal. But now he uses his hands, not to twist and bend iron or steel, but to ease twisted and bent limbs.

At our first meeting I watched him in action. Some of his patients went into a trance-like state as he moved among them. Later I interviewed about forty of the people he had treated. Many had suffered the agonies of arthritis and muscular complaints for years.

One woman could only move about by clinging to a metal frame. Another said she had been diagnosed by specialists as suffering from inoperable tumours. A 20-year-old secretary had lost her sight when she first sought Cain's help. Another patient told me he had a duodenal ulcer. And so it went on. All claimed they had been cured by John Cain. All were clearly telling the truth.

But as a journalist I had to establish that it was the real truth and not merely the truth of their own convictions. A person can suffer from headaches without it being migraine. A man with a heavy chill does not necessarily have bronchitis, despite what his doctor writes on his 'sick note'.

Also it is an established fact that many people who have suffered prolonged pain find relief simply by talking to others about their troubles. A sympathetic chat with someone who is obviously interested in their problem and is trying to help them can sometimes work wonders . . . temporarily. It is perhaps an indictment of our strained National Health Service that so many family doctors simply

8

do not have the time or the inclination to engage in cosy chats. Perhaps they have lost the art or maybe it is easier to write out a prescription for a bottle of pills.

I waited almost six months and then interviewed all the people again. I expected at least half of them to say "It seemed to work for a short time, but it didn't last."

To my amazement every person re-affirmed what they had told me six months earlier. In fact the majority said they felt even better.

The story of John Cain was published in the *News of the World* and the reader response was fantastic. For five days the office switchboard was jammed by callers all wanting the address and telephone number of John Cain. Letters arrived by every post. Thousands and thousands of them, all clamouring for information about John Cain. A secretary was employed full time dealing with the mountain of correspondence.

The story was picked up all over the world and even today I still get letters from Australia, New Zealand, parts of Africa and the West Indies asking to be put in touch with "The Healer".

When you think of it "The Healer" is not a bad title to be known by. You've got to earn it.

The days when people like John Cain were contemptuously dismissed by the medical profession as 'interfering amateurs' are thankfully drawing to a close. Today eminent scientists and psychologists – particularly in America, Russia, and certain European countries – are beginning to sit up and take note. Tentative investigations into the mystery of unorthodox healing have begun and John Cain has been the subject of an inquiry by several eminent physicians and scientists.

I have spoken to scientists, doctors, and churchmen who have met Cain and been intrigued by his methods and his success rate, particularly with arthritic ailments. All speak of his utter sincerity.

A vicar, whose wife was treated for a stiff arm by Cain, told me "He did her a lot of good after doctors had failed. There is an element of healing in all of us. In certain people, like John Cain, it is more developed." And he expressed the hope that enlightened medical bodies will take a more positive interest.

But it will be a long and slow process. If one fraction of the money spent on dishing out drugs to people who may not even require them could be channelled into investigating healing the pace could be dramatically increased.

My regret is that prejudice and partial paralysis of the official

9

medical mind will dictate otherwise.

Doctors, even those in Harley Street, do not claim to be able to cure the incurable. Neither do healers. If an optic nerve is destroyed nothing will restore sight to the affected eye. By the same token no Red Indian medicine man in the days of Custer's Last Stand would try to persuade someone who had survived a scalping that he could prescribe a miraculous hair restorer.

In this short introduction to the book about John Cain I have deliberately avoided entering into any discussion on the religious aspects of healing. I am a journalist, not a theologian. I deal in facts, not theories, and prefer to take the attitude of John Cain when he says "I don't know how it happens, but I know it does."

And after talking to many people – not just patients of John Cain – who have found relief at the hands of the Healer – I also know "It happens".

How Cain does it I don't pretend to know. People who have been treated by "The Healer" often speak of 'miracles'. It's a word that springs easily to the lips when a heavy blanket of excruciating pain is suddenly lifted and a dull November day seems like a May morning.

There is one 'minor miracle' though. How John Cain gets through his weekly work-load. Working as a blacksmith was easy by comparison. Every day there are people to be seen and treated, letters to answer, phone calls to take. Fortunately he is helped by a trusted band of friends and his devoted wife, Audrey. She never quibbled when he announced he was giving up his thriving business to become a healer.

"If he's happy that's all that matters" she told me.

I know that hundreds of John Cain's friends – and I count myself as one – will eagerly read this book and feel part of his work. I hope they will be joined by thousands more for this is a story of a man dedicated to helping others.

It is an insight into a remarkable man and when you finish the last page I know you will not be able to claim that you don't know John Cain.

# AUTHOR'S PREFACE

Writing this book about John Cain is, for me, a natural conclusion to a series of events in my own life. It is a pointer to the fact that he is a 'special' person and despite myself I have been directed towards him.

1975 was the year I first heard of him.

A friend said that her nephew was spending a lot of time with John Cain, the healer.

"His mother thinks it all a bit 'spooky'," she remarked.

"Oh, yes," I agreed, "he doesn't want to get too involved with people like that."

Four years on and well-used to seeing the man John Cain at work, never a day passes when I do not mention him to someone. Many a time the reaction of people is as mine was years ago and I smile each time I witness it.

To return to 1975. My teaching career was suddenly cut short because of redundancies in the profession. Being part-time, I was expendable.

I tried half-heartedly to get another post. But all suitable ones were too far away and I still had a young daughter of just two. It was difficult therefore to think about resuming my career for the time being.

About this time, the suspicions I had had about my daughter's slow progress were justified and it was diagnosed that she had brain-damage. Hospital visits to specialists and caring for her were to fill my days from now on.

Always a keen amateur writer, I wrote as an outlet for creative energy.

By 1977, I was writing features for the Liverpool Daily Post on a free-lance but regular basis.

A new career had been decided for me.

Working from home fitted in with my duties to my daughter and meant I could write at night if necessary.

In March, 1979, a friend, knowing I was always on the look-out for interesting people to write about informed me that John Cain, the healer, was going abroad soon.

"You'd better interview him quickly," she advised me.

Never one to turn down a good story I tore off to see him. He had moved from Eastham and now lived a stone's throw away from me. I did not connect him at all with the healer I'd had such misgivings about a few years earlier.

11

Being a journalist and interested in factual accuracy, I asked many searching questions. All the time I thought whilst talking to John Cain, 'well, you're very straight and I'm impressed by your humour, your sincerity, your confidence, and some of the case histories you're relating to me, but when *I* experience something, then I'll be truly interested.'

When he suggested I should receive a healing session, I agreed, although I confessed there wasn't much wrong with me a good week's holiday wouldn't cure.

One of his helpers and John Cain took me into a room with dimmed lights. I did not know what to expect.

Cain told me to close my eyes while he and his helper would relax me – a minor miracle in itself! After a few moments, and still conscious, I nevertheless felt relaxed. To my surprise, John Cain then said he felt directed to a painful spot on my spine, then to my right ankle which he thought, quite correctly, that I must have sprained at some time, then to a rheumy right thumb. The helper was massaging my left shoulder and he asked me if it was troublesome.

As it had been the reason for several visits to an osteopath the previous year who had suggested a 'hammer' to unlock the muscles, I could assure him it was!

I was impressed enough to go that same evening to a public healing session at the Civic Hall, Bromborough, where I was to interview several of John Cain's patients.

"Watch the 'beam-out'," he told me. It didn't really register with me what that was. But a few moments later I was amazed to see people dropping back like flies on to mattresses after Cain had stood at the front of the hall and merely raised his hands.

I wandered round the hall; not in the slightest bit inhibited. Nobody told me I should not talk to those waiting for treatment while a session was in progress. There was a distinct lack of formality and ceremony. You can be yourself here, I soon decided.

It was getting late. There were only a few mattresses left on the floor. I was anxious to see if I could experience this 'altered state of consciousness' I had heard so much about.

Knowing that I need not expect unconsciousness, I was more at ease. I closed my eyes and just floated for a few moments. Then someone took hold of my heels. I felt immediately a different sensation. My eye-lids felt as if leaden weights were on them and I felt compelled to laugh; a quiet, relaxed laugh which I could not prevent.

12

It was John Cain who had held my feet, I found out after.

I did not want to open my eyes. I told myself not to be stupid and to open them but they were stuck fast.

This lasted about ten minutes.

I knew I would have no difficulty at all in writing my article. I had seen enough and heard enough from the other people, whom, I reasoned, just could not all be making up the same story. Why should they? Their doctors and friends and families would surely have accused them by now of making up stories about their healing. In any case, some of them had already been the subject of a major investigation carried out by the *News of the World* and had agreed to have their names and addresses printed to testify to their cures.

I wrote my article for the Liverpool Daily Post – with no pain in my 'writing' thumb, by the way!

The response to the feature was unexpected but very gratifying.

Many hundreds of people wrote to or telephoned John Cain.

Some wrote letters to the newspaper.

Among the hundreds of letters were two abusive ones and the inevitable religious fanatic who believed that I had witnessed the 'work of the devil'. It is strange that the writers of such letters always camouflage as 'Christians', though they never seem to belong to a particular denomination or church.

However, a personal acquaintance, who does belong to a local church, spoke to me privately after reading my article in the paper. She expressed her doubts that an ordinary human being like John Cain should be carrying on 'healing like Jesus had done'.

I merely told her that John Cain was the last person to set himself up as some holy person or guru, and he certainly would never compare his work with that of Christ. But I could not resist reminding her of the criticism which had even been levelled at Jesus when he had healed the sick.

I don't ever enter into theological discussions; as a journalist I deal in straight facts, and I certainly had no intention of silencing my acquaintance with a clever response. But I seemed to have hit the right note; she admitted that she had never thought of healing outside the biblical context, and she had somehow quite overlooked the fact that even Jesus had been attacked for healing the sick.

Pat Sykes

Birkenhead
Merseyside

October 1979

13

# I

I grew increasingly interested in this man who lived virtually on my doorstep.

I read the first successful book written about him: "Heal, My Son!" and was fascinated by it. The journalist in me naturally wanted to follow up some of the people mentioned in it and see if they had received lasting benefit! But this had been done I soon discovered by the *News of the World* and *Reveille*.

For some time I had been interested in alternative medicine and here just around the corner from me was one of the busiest practitioners in existence of one branch of this medicine – healing!

Why wasn't there more known about him, I wondered?

As a journalist, I felt compelled to learn more. I was now quite convinced that he had a great contribution to offer to society.

So, I attended his sessions, as a journalist with my curiosity aroused and soon, also as a mother of a handicapped child.

I did not know or understand how John Cain might help my daughter but then neither does he admit to understanding how the healing takes place. Somehow, if she could be helped, then I felt confident that John Cain was the person to do it. And certainly, there was nothing to be lost since so little is known about brain-damage.

I soon realised that John Cain is an enigma; an ordinary man on the one hand, on the other, a healer with an extraordinary gift. He is most definitely a positive and extrovert character and as such attracts attention; but he does not dominate a room with clever argument. He leaves theorising to others. When he speaks about healing, he does so with authority. He dominates rather by sheer personality; he is tough, uncompromising yet compassionate and dedicated. Somehow, when you meet John Cain in a crowded room he stands out, even when he is silent. His presence makes itself felt.

John Cain has had his critics; he is a frank and open character who ignores the subtleties of diplomatic speech and who acts as he feels like, totally disregarding that some people don't like to learn the truth.

His critics must be seen in perspective; their number is very small but they are vociferous within that limited circle in which they operate.

It would be foolish and totally out of perspective if they were given undue prominence; on the other hand, it would be equally foolish not to mention them at all. The amazing fact which emerges when one investigates the criticism levelled against John Cain is that none of his critics have as much hinted that Cain's healing powers were in doubt. On the contrary, several of his most vociferous critics testify that they or close relatives had been helped by him, often in circumstances where doctors had literally given up hope for the patient.

It has always been events which happened *after* John Cain had helped them that caused anger, frustration and ultimately unpleasant noises.

Once John Cain had helped them or their relatives, they were so grateful and emotionally overcome by the experience, that they offered to become 'helpers'. These are dedicated men and women who assist John Cain, especially during meetings where hundreds of patients attend at the same time.

But the truth is that they did not really want to 'help' John Cain, they wanted to manage him.

When I first started writing about John Cain and observed him during healing sessions and also his healer-patient relationship I realised immediately that he was not only totally different from what I expected a healer to be like but I actually thought that he was probably very naïve.

But I also realised that my journalistic experience had taught me to expect behaviour from the healer which was 'typical' and in keeping with the practices of healers in general.

John Cain's personality, his unspoiled, natural behaviour and especially his defiance of other people's opinion about what he should do and what he should not do, set him apart from other healers. Cain is not interested in canvassing public approval and he cannot abide sycophantic 'hangers-on'.

For example, some of his helpers were furious with Cain for being too friendly with other patients, when to be otherwise would be totally unnatural to him. Deep down, there was just simple jealousy that Cain should have spent more time with others than with them. Unfortunately, whenever they tried to change John Cain, they chose arguments which were hurtful, not to Cain but to the other patients.

Some of the 'helpers' criticised him for wasting time and energy visiting patients in hospital who had only a few days or weeks to live.

16

"They are going to die anyway; why waste your time on them with healing? It is bound to end in failure!"

This criticism really angered John Cain because for him there is no such thing as failure in healing. If he can help a person to die peacefully and without pain, then he has achieved all he attempted to do. Too many simple-minded people equate the word 'healing' with 'cure'.

Others were trying to 'manage' John Cain; they hoped that their influence on him might help towards greater fame. They argued that he should do what other healers did: give an allotted time to patients, wear a white coat, do this, that and the other. It is strange that they never saw how much John Cain disliked being categorised with others. He went on being just John Cain.

Criticism against John Cain has been very limited, and it would be fair to say that it has only taken place on a parochial level. My research showed four former helpers who had written between them about forty letters to local newspapers. Seen in perspective, especially on a national level, you may wonder why I even mentioned those 'helpers'.

I have done so because they did influence John Cain in some respects. Today he is far more careful when allowing a person to become a 'helper'. "I have learned my lesson," he told me, "I know now how important it is for helpers to rid themselves of their personal ego. They must know that they can only help if they allow themselves to be channels for my healing gift as much as I am a channel for those who work through me. 'Helpers' can only be of benefit to me and those who come for healing, if they keep a low profile and don't try to run the healing session. I act and move as the spirit moves me; if I feel that a particular patient needs my attention, I give it to him or her and I don't intend ever going round with a stop watch in order not to offend those who believe, mistakenly, that they are entitled to the same number of minutes."

The second group of critics, again from a limited circle and small in number but vociferous, object to John Cain on different grounds. John Cain has in the past belonged to Spiritualist Churches and he has also been, for a while, a member of the *National Federation of Spiritual Healers*. He left this organisation because he thought the Federation gives out memberships and certificates too easily and without investigating healing methods thoroughly enough. At his own demonstration for admittance into the Federation, he thought it farcical that he was asked to treat some of the healers who themselves belonged to the Federation. 'How can so many sick people treat other sick people?' was his main criticism. Furthermore, he deplores the practice of wearing white coats employed by many of the Federation's certificate holders.

Cain has never been afraid of speaking his mind; he is uncompromisingly frank and he never camouflages the truth as he sees it. Even those 'hard-line' critics from within the organisations admit that John Cain has never waited until he was some safe distance away from those whom he spoke out against but that he always stood up and challenged those whom he considered 'engaging in phoney practices and exploiting the public'. None of the critics from within those organisations has ever suggested or implied that John Cain is not the great healer he has become known as. On the contrary, my research has shown that even his severest critics admit that his gift of healing is phenomenal. They do object though that this gift should be in the hands of a man who does not conform to their way of thinking.

"I have broken with organised Spiritualist centres mainly because of the standard of mediumship and healing," says John Cain. "I have seen little evidence of any worth from those platforms of Spiritualist gatherings to which I was invited. But I have seen some dreadful healing sessions. I thought they were an insult to the intelligence of those poor people who had gone there to get relief from pain or healing.

"One in particular sticks out in my mind. It was in a Spiritualist church in North Wales. I saw one healer, supposedly in a trance and talking to patients who called her 'doctor'. I've seen thousands of people in trance-state and should know what it looks like and I reckon she was never in trance.

"Anyway, she went over to another 'healer', (I don't know what the patient's condition was, by the way, it could have been depression, for all I know!) and said, 'you push down and I'll take it away from his stomach'. Then she snatched at his stomach with her hands and appeared to throw something down on the floor five or six times. I'd had enough and just said to her, 'the way you're going on, you'll contaminate the carpet' and I walked out, disgusted."

John Cain also deplores the practice amongst some healers of wearing white coats and masquerading as medically-qualified doctors. But even worse than this, he believes, is the sickening sight of such healers washing their hands in prepared bowls after dealing with each patient.

18

"I refuse to be a part of such practices," says Cain, indignantly. "It is insulting and offensive to the patients, for a start. If a patient has a contagious condition I would not dream of treating them with other members of the public, but see them privately."

Cain recalls spending a week listening to lectures and demonstrations of healing and mediumship at Stanstead.

"By the end of the week," he says, "I'd seen nothing to convince me that anyone there had any special gifts. Then came one of the worst exhibitions I've ever seen.

"Several people were invited to give demonstrations of healing methods. One man, in his late 60's, was supposed to be in a trance and was guided round the patients by his wife, shouting out directions. He approached one patient and began asking her, 'can you feel heat? Is this where the pain is? Can you feel tingling?' To all of these questions, she replied 'no'.

"I knew she had a throat condition because I'd treated her earlier in the week. He touched every part of her body except her throat! Then he staggered forward like a drunk, threw one arm into the air and stabbed at the air with his fist and grunted three times. Then his wife shouted, 'don't any of you people recognise whose this voice is?' They all shouted back, 'no'. She told them: 'It's Frank! It's Frank!' So everybody joined in, 'God Bless Frank!'

"Frank was supposed to be a former well-known Spiritualist who had died."

At another such course at Stanstead in 1975, Cain incurred the displeasure of the organisers who maintained that "John Cain has flouted the rules and regulations because he healed at the wrong times"! He was accused of moving chairs and cushions for the patients' use in the wrong place, and for good measure, one of the critics added that "Cain's ashtray was always filled by ten o'clock in the morning."

It is when Cain is in the company of others who claim to be healers that he stands out most. It is obvious that he cannot abide the formalities and ceremonies attached to these healing sessions. One can see how he becomes impatient and brusque – to the point of rebellion almost, when these ceremonies and rules interfere with his healing work.

When Cain feels that someone is in need of healing, he will give it, "anywhere and at any time", he asserts. It is his blunt replies to those who put ceremonies, rules and showbiz first and healing second, which often provoke the criticism of those whom Cain considers

19

'perhaps well intentioned but misguided'.

Fred Curtis, a Spiritualist platform speaker from Nottinghamshire, encountered Cain for the first time at that particular healing course at Stanstead. "I did not agree with Cain's strong criticism," he recalls, "but I could see that he had been subjected to interference in his healing work right through the week. Cain should have been given more time to demonstrate his unique healing gifts.

"To my mind, anything new should be fully investigated and not dismissed because people don't understand it, as was the case with Cain during that week. I have not seen all the healers at work in Great Britain, but many, and to the best of my knowledge, John Cain is the best yet."

It is a matter of record that none of the criticism levelled against Cain concerns his remarkable healing gift and his extraordinary successes. His critics don't like his forthright speech, they object to his blunt criticism of themselves, they consider him irreverent, unrefined and common. They believe that his first duty is to the rules and regulations and not the sick who come to him for healing.

John Cain knows full well that he has not endeared himself to the Spiritualist movement by his outspokenness but he is unafraid of its censure and will continue to expose phoney practitioners. As he says: "Spiritualism is all right; it's some of the spiritualists who are the trouble!"

John Cain is very outspoken when he talks about mediums and healers. "I can only acknowledge a mere handful of good mediums in this country," he says. "As far as healers go, I have personally only ever known one, Harry Edwards, who had that true gift of healing. There are obviously others, but I have never met them in those churches and on those platforms."

Cain is often criticised for his life-style. He still enjoys his drink, speaks plainly as he has always done (being John Cain, he has not developed a phoney way of talking, so common among spiritualists); he has an impish, flirtatious way with women – in fact, he is still basically the tough army P.T. instructor, the blacksmith in a shipyard, the successful self-made business-man.

"Just look at him with a cigarette in his mouth, whilst healing," was the carp from two 'healers' at Stanstead.

John Cain remembers the occasion well.

"I was having a drink and smoking at the bar opposite these two, when a girl called over to me to lift her headache. I laid on the hands and the pain went. Then came the comment. I replied, 'Yes, but I can' and hoped this hit them where I aimed it, right at their own inability to heal."

This open lack of modesty could easily be misinterpreted as egotism or plain big-headedness. To John Cain, it is manifestation of the confidence he has in himself and in the higher intelligence which works through him. A confidence which is essential to him to carry out his work, he believes.

There have been some strange reactions by the media to John Cain's personality. Some journalists have gone so far as to portray him as Liverpool's answer to Rasputin!

After the *News of the World* article appeared in Britain, an Arabic newspaper copied it, adding a beard to make him look more sinister. This brought the secretary of a Sheik to John Cain's door bearing gifts; a crate of whisky and hundreds of cigarettes because he thought this was what was expected of him after reading the 'translated' article.

John Cain the healer and John Cain the man are the same person; he could not achieve such successful healing, I feel certain, if he attempted to change.

That would be a strain on him. And it is his relaxed manner which is so important to his rapport with his patients.

Anyone who has sat opposite a stern-faced G.P. or a brilliant but out-of-reach specialist and felt a 'bag of nerves' will know how stressful it is to have to talk about what is after all a very personal and important thing to you, your own body!

Many people go so far as to write a list of what is wrong with them in case they are so tongue-tied they'll forget. This is not to say that there are no sympathetic doctors, or specialists. But the increased growth in drug manufacture has meant that world-wide medical care seems to be moving further away from the humanitarian treatment of the patient and is more geared to a scientific approach.

A frightening thought.

John Cain presents no awesome figure to his 'friends', as he soon calls his patients. Though he can be irritated by time-wasters and ditherers.

Patients who want to go into his centre together, and fuss about having to wait for friends receive a sharp reminder that they are wasting valuable time and disturbing the peaceful atmosphere.

John Cain is many things to many people.

For me, he personifies the phrase 'brotherhood of man' more than any person I have met.

I have always found it difficult, if not impossible, to write articles about John Cain for newspapers and present him to my readers objectively and as he really is. There is never enough space for an 'in-depth' article which allows a real profile story. Besides, editors and readers are more interested in John Cain's phenomenal healing successes.

Meeting John Cain has been a memorable experience for me as it has been for many thousands of people. Well-known reporters and journalists of national newspapers who had come originally to write about him, and some who came to debunk him if that should prove possible, have become his friends. Journalists, like policemen, do not make friends lightly and easily. They know the danger to their profession.

I acknowledge John Cain without the embarrassment I would feel for, say, an evangelical preacher or the fear that to know or see him at work makes me an extremist or a fanatical follower. I have never been one to embrace causes too readily, chiefly because their ideals, whilst purporting to benefit mankind, end up being the more important and often make worthless and cheap the greatest gift mankind has, life itself.

I do not understand how his healing works or why he should have been selected to be a channel for healing. I do know that he can heal and I hope that the accounts in this book related to me by the many grateful and genuine people who have received help at his hands, will give cheer to others for whom the phrase, 'there is nothing more we can do for you' means a life of agonising pain.

There is something more that can be done for you.

And the man, John Cain, will prove it to you.

# II

Since John Cain first made the headlines in British newspapers in 1972, journalists have tried to give their readers a picture of the man which would do justice to him and his extraordinary gift of healing.

As in a cartoon, certain characteristics were exaggerated so as to give him a 'build-up' which would contrast sharply with the expected and the usual. Of course, there is much of the unexpected and unusual in John Cain, but it is fair to say that some of the descriptions which were given of him were heavily loaded and bordered more on the sensational than on reality.

I mentioned earlier the incident following an article which appeared in an Arabic 'translation' of Alan Whittaker's report in the *News of the World*. But exaggerations about John Cain are very common in all newspapers. I can understand this quite well because he does not conform to an expected pattern of behaviour. We are so accustomed to associating a healer with some esoteric, slightly eccentric and often *holier-than-thou* character, that meeting John Cain must come as a surprise, and to many as a shock.

This is largely due to his refusal to change and to adopt a personality which is alien to him. Cain has remained the same Liverpudlian lad he has always been. He speaks as he spoke before he took up healing and he has not changed his life style either. That is to say he only changed that which was inevitable. For example, before becoming a full-time healer, he was a successful blacksmith with his own business.

The yard stick with which a successful, self-made man measures his progress, is sometimes the type of car he drives. John Cain used to drive a Rolls Royce. And bearing in mind that he then had an annual income of about £20,000, he was about twenty times better off than the average wage earner at that time. A Rolls Royce does not go unnoticed in the area where John Cain used to live. Similarly, John liked his drink at the local and his regular evenings out with friends. There was a Rolls Royce outside, but he was still the same man as he had always been. Those familiar with the Liverpudlian dialect know that the language is down-to-earth. 'Swearing' in Liverpool is not the same as using the same words in the South. The invocation of members of the Holy Family, which might be interpreted as 'blaspheming' in refined Southern circles, is in Liverpool a very common occurence. After all, there are plenty of Irish immigrants in Liverpool who would be struck dumb overnight if the use of holy names were to be outlawed!

Few healers, if any at all, who become successful and can lay claim to extraordinary happenings, would remain on their home patch. They would probably be obsessed with the idea of moving to London and setting up some impressive healing sanctuary. They feel that they have to learn good bedside manners because that would be expected of them. They learn how to flatter hypochondriacs, and most of all, they learn what to charge for their 'services'. Those, who become well known, like Harry Edwards, are treated almost as Gurus by their followers.

No doubt, John Cain has been a fly in the ointment of Spiritual Healing since his name first appeared in newspapers. In the opinion of those who had worked hard to build up an aura of refinement and piety, Cain was a disgrace, a country bumpkin who drank, smoked and used bad language.

What they most objected to was that John Cain always spoke his mind and did not mince his words. When he wanted a drink, he did not quietly slip out of his 'sanctuary' and hit the bottle, but he shared his drink with those who wanted one. His less refined nostrils probably preferred the smoke of cigarettes to that incense which is often found in those pseudo-pious establishments where healing takes place.

Reporters and journalists from many national newspapers, who themselves are used to hard drink, a good smoke and plain language, liked that man. Whilst investigating his work with the same thoroughness as they had investigated other healers, they considered John Cain's life style worthy of mention.

And so the legend about Cain grew with each new article that appeared. Looking through the thousands of column inches which have been written about him, as much space is given to describing John in contrast to other healers' life styles as has been given to his work.

John Cain's life before he became a healer was in no way extraordinary or exceptional enough to merit special mention. He was successful, but in comparison with many other Liverpudlians who have made headlines in newspapers – the Beatles, comedians like Ken

Dodd, Jimmy Tarbuck and Tom O'Connor – Cain's rise to prosperity was very modest.

He was born in Chester on the twenty-first of April, 1931. His father was a postman and because of his job, the family moved to Bromborough, Merseyside, where Cain attended the local village school.

Cain went on to attend Woodslea Secondary school which he left at the age of fourteen.

After a brief spell at Lever Brothers, Port Sunlight, he began his apprenticeship as a blacksmith at Cammell Laird's shipyard, Birkenhead.

Cain began his National Service, ten days after his twenty-first birthday and on completion of the initial ten weeks' training, went on a course to qualify as an army P.T. instructor.

This was a natural choice for Cain, a keen sportsman, especially in the field of Judo.

After the army, Cain returned to the shipyard, was married in 1956 to Audrey, the same year he started up his own business. They had two children, John jnr., now aged twenty-three and Janette, now aged twenty-one.

Of course, most people who go to a healer or read about healing find it difficult to reconcile Cain's ordinary background and natural behaviour with the extraordinary success as a healer and his amazing gifts. I agree that it is difficult to put him into the right perspective, and that difficulty accounts largely for that new picture which has emerged: John Cain the enigma.

After eight months of observing John Cain at close quarters, I have come to realise that the enigma is really the healer and not the man. He himself cannot explain his gifts, and because these gifts show themselves in all manner of phenomena and unexpected results, one never ceases to ask the questions: 'what is he?' 'what is he doing this time?' and even, 'who is he?'.

As far as I am concerned, and I believe that all my journalist colleagues apply the same criteria, the proof of the pudding is in the eating!

If a person is really ill and the doctors can no longer do anything but prescribe sedatives and powerful pain killers, and if that person's health is improved or even restored by the ex-blacksmith, John Cain, then I have something to write about. I doubt whether the most learned scientific minds can explain what has really happened. As far as an investigative journalist is concerned, three points matter: first, it must be established that the person was really as sick as he or she claimed. This can easily be ascertained by making the right enquiries in the right quarters. Secondly it must be shown beyond any doubt that the person's health has improved and sometimes been restored; I go further and suggest that such an improvement should be a long-term one. Again, there are ways and means of finding that out. Thirdly, I want to know whether this improvement was brought about by a man without any medical qualifications and without the use of drugs.

If I am satisfied on all three counts, I believe I can tell my readers that I have witnessed a modern-day miracle!

During the last few months, I have seen many of those miracles; and so have many of my colleagues. We all have written about them and told the public in our respective newspapers. But there is a limit of space, even for such good news . . . or should I say especially for 'good news'.

Having put John Cain, the man, into perspective, I shall now attempt to give an account of his healing. Time and time again, John's way of thinking comes through.

It is impossible to divorce the man from his achievements completely. Some of the extraordinary happenings take place in an environment which, in my opinion, must influence Cain's actions. For example, when he attends functions where so-called 'healers' are in abundance, and where he feels sickened at the sight of what they are doing, John Cain's reaction is one of righteous indignation. He gives healing almost in defiance of the circus which is going on around him.

Come to think of it, I believe I have seen John Cain carry out healing several times 'in anger' or when reacting against something which he considered phoney and even evil. Such events are always more dramatic than the usual, tranquil and very peaceful healing sessions. But if you want to get to know John Cain a little better, it is important to see it all.

I am not so much concerned with the chronological sequence of John Cain's work than with the variety of case histories. Several extraordinary healing successes have already been described in the paperback 'HEAL, MY SON!', which was published in 1977. But that was only the beginning.

# III

In April, 1978, John Cain, his wife, Audrey and their son, John and daughter, Janette, left their modern bungalow in Eastham and moved into a rambling Edwardian house in North Road, Birkenhead.

The decision to move had come about indirectly through a healing.

John Cain had been visiting a child patient in North Road. As he left the house, one day, he saw the 'For Sale' sign outside number 20.

"I'm having that house," he said with certainty.

He knew the interior of this type of house and felt it would fulfil some of his ambitions. For instance, he had wanted for a while to do fewer public sessions and work more from home. His present bungalow was limited in space and it had reached the stage where his son's bedroom was converted daily into a healing room.

Also, John Cain had always wanted a gymnasium or a games room at the rear of his home and this place seemed to him ideal.

Cain was so certain about the move that he even predicted accurately who would buy their bungalow.

"He's not a young man," he announced to his family. "And he is lame in one leg." That was exactly so!

The sale negotiations were completed in just over a month which surprised everyone concerned.

They moved and the house was turned upside down whilst being modernised. All the time, of course, the healing continued, at Bromborough Civic Centre and at other halls.

The house is now comfortable and well-modernised and the Healing Centre, not John Cain's gymnasium, exactly, is well and truly opened.

Some of John Cain's dedicated patients and friends made contributions towards the centre and its building went through without a single hitch.

Living in North Road makes administration duties much easier for John's wife, Audrey, who works tirelessly for the centre. She has an office where she answers the hundreds of letters received weekly asking for help and information about her husband.

There is always a pile of letters to be posted on her desk and always stamps to be licked – not everyone thinks of sending stamped-addressed envelopes!

There are telephones all over the house and whatever room Audrey Cain is in she cannot escape from them. Always her tone is polite, helpful; although she must repeat the same phrases over and over again . . . "yes, John will see you. Just come along . . . "

But she enjoys seeing so many sick people receiving benefit from the healing and although the strain on both John and Audrey Cain's life at times is great – their social life is very limited – she bears up and continues to support her husband.

Miss Ethel Humphreys was healed by John Cain a few years ago when she suffered from painful arthritis. She became a great friend and is now in charge of organising Cain's public sessions at Bromborough Civic Hall and the daily group healings at John Cain's house.

She is there at the door with a smile of welcome and advice to newcomers on the procedure, which is precious little really, because informality is the key-note.

There are no awkward introductions: 'Won't I have to tell Mr Cain all about my complaint? What about my medical history, and the drugs I'm taking?' are the questions which seem to worry people most.

But no-one is expected to say anything if they don't want to. Ethel writes down a patient's complaint on a card which is handed to a helper in the centre.

Already the Healing Centre has become a Mecca for the sick and disabled and at least fifty to eighty patients a day from all over the area and other parts of Great Britain tread the path to the centre. Many more patients from abroad are making special visits, and in the course of two weeks, whilst working on this book, I met and interviewed several from Europe and overseas.

Cain's whole life is healing and he is often unable to switch off from his work.

He has the strong desire to see people well and the only way he can do this is by allowing it to spill over into his private life; the danger then is that it can dominate all else.

John Cain is mindful of this but on the other hand, he does not ever feel he can turn anyone away. Of course, he would be less than human if he never admitted to tiredness and exhaustion.

28

Cain had recognised that his son, John, Jnr. is developing as a healer and he now works full-time assisting his father.

Offers have come John Cain's way to take up a new life in America and Canada where he could live in the lap of luxury. They offer enormous fees in those countries from just one night's healing session.

But Cain is not interested in that.

Similarly Cain has turned down offers from promoters who want to organise large theatrical performances all over Britain.

"I am very settled on Merseyside," he says. "I will never leave here. And after all, what is 'big' money? I have all I want for myself and my family."

# IV

In the early stages of John Cain's work as a healer, it was stated by two independent, highly-respected mediums that Cain's controlling spirit guide is a Dr Carl Heindrich Hoffman who had lived in Austria.

Later, John Cain himself also acknowledged that he had Japanese and Chinese guides who strongly influenced his healing. People had testified that on occasions, Carl had materialised in Cain's place; at other times Cain's features had taken on an oriental aspect.

Cain was healing successfully by the laying on of hands, until one memorable day in 1973 when he discovered that his healing was to move in another direction.

He was treating a patient who had had a hysterectomy. She was seated on a stool and he placed one hand on her stomach whilst the other worked slowly down her spinal column.

Cain had closed his eyes, as was usual for concentration in the healing. When he opened them later, he was astounded to see that the girl patient had bent right back over from the waist, a seemingly impossible position for her condition. He felt he had been in a trance-like state and she also.

From this point on, patients he treated would frequently go into what was best described as 'an altered state of consciousness'. Some of them in this state would self-manipulate limbs with amazing agility whilst Cain himself did not even touch them and could stand back and observe. In retrospect, he now recognises this development in the healing as direct intervention by 'spirit guides' to speed up the healing process. Some patients with extremely painful and stiffened limbs could begin manipulation from the very first session whereas previously, Cain may have had to work on them for several sessions before they felt able to move with any freedom and agility.

Though from now it always appeared that his patients went into the altered state of consciousness whilst Cain apparently remained fully conscious, it was established by interested scientists who measured his brain-wave patterns, that during the healing, Cain registered a 'very high alpha state' and also his heartbeat was five times higher than the patients'.

Hypnosis was suggested as playing a large part in inducing the altered state in patients. Cain readily admits he has an interest in hypnosis but the observer can soon ascertain that there are no suggestive practices involved. And indeed I can personally vouch that this is not the case. In fact, John Cain may be standing at the side or even behind a patient so that no eye contact is possible. Nothing is said; Cain does not need to talk but allows himself to be a passive channel for the spirit healers to work through.

John Cain is convinced that his healing is progressive and that his 'spirit guides' are continually experimenting with his patients, and evolving new healing methods.

Over the last twelve months he has begun to develop the use of acupressure points to assist in the healing. Over 5,000 years old, this method of oriental origin, Cain believes, is manifestation of 'Eastern guides' at work.

Cain located these pressure points without previous referral to books on the subject. His later research confirmed that he was one hundred per cent accurate in his location of them.

John Cain has always been able to 'pick-up' trouble spots on a patient's body even when the patient is unaware he had anything wrong! At one time, Cain says that he felt his hands were directed to these areas and though this can still happen, Cain is discovering that some 'intelligence' will often now reveal to him in other ways where a patient is in need of healing.

A patient can, whilst in the altered state, direct Cain to a painful area by even the slightest of self-manipulations. Once, Cain tells of a man who had not written down a back condition on his card because he had attended the session for another complaint. Cain surprised him after this session by informing him that his lower back was in need of healing because the man had manipulated both thighs when Cain had merely held his ankles!

In my observations, I have also witnessed a patient who had lost the ability to write because of nerve paralysis, touching his shoulder repeatedly whilst in the altered state. This immediately indicated to John Cain that this was a trouble spot neither he nor the patient had yet realised was in need of healing.

Although John Cain maintains that he is no theorist it is quite obvious that he gives much thought to what happens in the healing processes. He has formulated his own theories based on the various phenomena which occur.

31

He is very cautious, however, about making pronouncements until he is absolutely certain of his facts.

For instance, one patient talked about pressure points being indented during 'absent healing'. Cain received confirmation very soon that this was not just an isolated case as within days several other patients confirmed that this had taken place with them also.

In the same way he has ascertained over the years that there is definite proof of what he terms 'pain dispersal'.

Unlike other healers, he does not agree that there are no side effects from healing and that what can happen to a patient's body after healing is a sure way of testifying that something has taken place within the body and healing has indeed started.

"If a patient comes with an arthritic shoulder," Cain explains, "their movement can be very limited. Sometimes, after healing, they will experience relief from pain and freedom in that shoulder. They can feel marvellous. Then the next day or even days after, they may experience extreme pain, not in the shoulder, but all over the body. This is a sign that the deposits lodged in the shoulder joint have begun to disperse into the system. It is very important that patients realise this as sometimes they have been in agony and have not returned. Their healing then has not been completed.

"Some patients feel a nuisance and will not contact me if they have a set-back, but I would prefer they telephoned me or wrote to me rather than suffer in silence."

Sometimes, just speaking to Cain strengthens the link and the healing, which may have halted temporarily, starts up again. Cain has heard some patients say that they are taking up his valuable time when there are others worse than they. But as he says: "No condition is too trivial – a rheumatic thumb which prevents someone from doing their job properly needs healing just as much as a really bad arthritic shoulder."

Since the first occasion when a patient went into the altered state, Cain has tried to puzzle out why various phenomena occur. For instance, patients have been known to get up and dance or demonstrate judo and karate movements. Cain himself was a keen dancer and interested in yoga and judo. He is of the belief now that what he has been and done in the past is somehow reflected in his patients' reactions whilst in the altered state.

To those who would argue that dancing or judo have nothing to do with healing, Cain has his answer. If a patient is very shy and inhibited, in addition to being physically ill, then 'movement' whilst

32

in the altered state can release tensions which, if not released, might even delay the process of physical healing with some patients.

John Cain feels that over the years he has learned to detect those who are not going to respond well to treatment. He is not talking about sceptics, because he has healed many of those! But he thinks that in just the same way as some people have been known to say, 'I'm going to die' only for it to be written on their tombstones, 'I told you so!', John Cain has met some people who were too miserable to want to get well and who seemed to revel in their dispirited frame of mind.

Whilst John Cain feels most unhappy to refuse treatment to anybody, I have seen two of such cases myself and I consider John's reactions to these persons important enough to explain it. As I have said, they are usually not what might be termed 'sceptics'. On the contrary, the gentleman I saw claimed to be a 'healer' himself and a Spiritualist, though he admitted that his 'healing' left much to be desired.

But it was obvious, not only to John Cain, that this man would have been very miserable indeed, had he been freed from the illnesses and symptoms he claimed to suffer from.

The man's wife was obviously sick, but they both lived in a world of drama and exaggeration. They were more concerned with the room in which John worked, commenting on the lack of paintings of spirit guides, talking about their own Spirit communicators, than allowing John Cain to give them healing.

Cain became obviously irritated, and he soon made it plain that he was not going to waste his time on useless chatter, though I am quite sure that idle chatter was probably their only purpose for the visit.

Over the last two years, Cain has seen an increasing amount of the use of aggression by some patients in the healing sessions. They will slap and bang the floor and appear quite fierce! Cain thinks this is as beneficial as the laughing, crying, shaking and dancing which many patients do whilst in the altered state.

Their aggression can sometimes be turned against him but neither he nor any of his patients have ever been hurt in any of these sessions.

In the same way, great love can be shown to Cain by patients, both men and women, and he sees this as a natural release of emotions all-important to their 'whole' healing.

Of all the aspects of John Cain's healing perhaps the one most difficult to explain is 'Absent Healing'.

This can take place literally hundreds of miles away and there have been many letters written to John Cain by people puzzled and amazed at the healing they have received from a distance. Absent Healing can happen in a variety of ways.

On one occasion, whilst sitting in John Cain's lounge and talking to him about this book I intended to write, a telephone call came through from Ireland. It was from a telephone-box; hardly conducive to a healing session with the constant threat of being interrupted by pips!

However, quite unperturbed, John Cain directed the caller, who had just read an article about Cain and had never heard of him before, to make the sick person comfortable in a chair. Cain further asked the caller to put his hands on the two trouble-spots of the sick person – the throat and stomach – and he, Cain would link-up with the patient.

The pips went and that was that. Five minutes later the 'phone went again. It was the Irishman reporting that the pains had disappeared! Too late, I realised I should have leapt to my feet to get the name and address. However, there are testimonies galore in Cain's files, and he assured me there would be plenty of names I could follow up any time.

A later chapter will deal with some stories about Absent Healing.

The use of John Cain's photograph to help in the linking-up has proved a phenomenal success. "Some people go into a trance looking at anything," was the comment made by a psychiatrist who discussed the practice of healing with Cain's photograph in a *News of the World* article, following the major investigation of Cain by that paper.

Yet, there have been too many extraordinary occurrences to allow this aspect to be dismissed with a glib comment.

There have been reports of unusual heat-waves emanating from the photograph; stories of marks both on the body and on the photograph when it had been placed against a painful area.

I have tested the photograph myself and discovered that my eyes lose focus after a few seconds. I blink but normal focus does not return and before long a heavy drowsiness takes over. I experimented with other photographs and have not felt any different, so that I can only report that Cain's photograph works for me.

Publishers refuse on principle to get involved with controversial subjects they consider for publication. Perhaps it is significant that an incident with John Cain's photograph made an unexpected but profound impression on my publisher.

A Director from another publishing house happened to pick up a photograph of John Cain; within seconds, and quite unpremeditated, the gentleman suddenly slumped back in his seat and found himself in a strange state of total relaxation. When he came out of this state, after about three minutes, he declared himself totally reinvigorated and feeling as fresh as he might feel after a holiday.

The point my publisher made was that his colleague would never have allowed himself to appear gullible or impressionable in his presence. After all, such an incident breaks through the poker-face relationship so common among publishers.

Meditation on an object in Yoga is common practice and helps clear the mind. Meditating on John Cain's photograph appears to have the same effect and it can also produce heat and relieve pain as many people have testified. That is something which experts have not explained and glib comments do not give a satisfactory answer.

Much as Cain would like, he just cannot make the many house visits he is asked to do. For this reason, he believes that he can 'condition' a member of a family or a relation to enable them to help the sick person who is unable to visit his centre.

Cain explained it to me:

"The conditioning may be done by telephoning; I will instruct the caller to lay on hands whilst I link-up with them. There have been many reports of successful healing done this way. I may suggest, if I think it will help even more, that the relative comes to the centre. There I'll put him or her into the altered state of consciousness and the spiritual side takes over. In many cases, the desire to help the sick person at home is heightened and I've found very few people this hasn't worked with.

"There is a danger that those I have 'conditioned' may come to believe that they have developed a healing power. In such cases, I can detect when the ego has become overblown and it is found that they can no longer assist the sick person beneficially."

Cain has a highly-developed clairvoyant gift which he could use all the time, if he so wished. His healing work is more important to him, however. But there are occasions, when quite by chance he will find himself in a healing session giving information to a patient which he obviously gained clairvoyantly. There is always a reason for this and it is always relevant to the healing process. For instance, a patient may be hiding from Cain some emotional or traumatic experience which has caused them to be ill in the first place.

John Cain has many times picked this up. He also thinks that his 'guides' direct him to use this gift when the patient is in need of real help but has strong doubts about healing being successful.

Cain may, for example, reveal to them exactly when they became ill or had an accident. This demonstration of clairvoyance is often just what is needed to break down the patient's apprehensions and doubts. The healing can then begin.

John Cain is convinced that he can foresee quite some time ahead how his healing will develop. It is a constantly changing process and he believes that in time there will be less laying on of hands involved in the healing.

About this he says, "My confidence in the 'spirit intelligence' is growing all the time. Because the number of patients coming to me increases daily, my work-load gets heavier and I cannot always get round to everyone.

"The 'intelligence' realises this and feels the healing must continue with less contact.

"Psychologically, though, many patients expect and need contact and it will never be withheld from those in need."

# V

I have selected thirty three case histories from many more I investigated during my research. The choice was mine entirely, and I selected these cases because each of them appears to me typical of many similar healing examples by John Cain.

All the patients of John Cain whom I interviewed agreed readily to have their story published, and none of them expressed a preference for remaining anonymous.

Several cases have been edited by me insofar as I deleted occurrences during the healing sessions which were of an obviously psychic nature. I felt that the psychic phenomena experienced by some of the patients and related by them, might complicate the narrative; I deliberately concentrated on healing alone.

I sincerely hope that I have been able to convey the spontaneity of the interviews, though I am regretfully aware that it is impossible to share with my readers that aura of happiness and gratefulness to John Cain which permeated every interview.

## 1.

"You have multiple sclerosis. This is a very serious disease but I will try and help you."

These were the words John Cain spoke to ERIC DAVIES of Willaston, Wirral, when he first came to a healing session in November, 1977.

Eric was impressed by Cain's positive and confident approach and decided to attend for six months to give the healing therapy a chance. After all, nothing medically had helped in all those years and the doctors, baffled by the disease, could only prescribe tranquillisers.

Eric had come to a crisis point in 1977. Previously a very keen sportsman, he had not given in easily to the change in his body and had fought it since 1959. Now, he felt he was fighting a losing battle.

He had deterioriated to the extent where walking was an effort and his general health was very poor.

He was very sceptical when he first went to Cain, and only observed the first time. At the second session, Eric lay down and remarked afterwards to Cain that he'd never experienced such relaxation ever before in his life.

Although the onlooker might comment that Eric, still walking with the aid of a stick and having poor balance, does not seem to have progressed very far he feels this is not the case:

"Since attending Cain," he says, "my condition has been stabilized. I have suffered no serious set-backs in those months such as dizziness; poor vision; leg pains; stomach disorders; lack of energy; all of which were common before. My attitudes have changed, both spiritually and mentally. I have been able to keep my job which calls for much decision-making and deal with work pressures more calmly.

"I have more control over my limbs than I have had for years."

Eric is very pleased he made the decision to visit John Cain and also that he carried on seeing him after the six months trial period was up.

"I am confident," he says, "that the treatment will continue and my complaint will be healed. I can't stress enough the importance of the relaxation I gain from John Cain's sessions. Although I've never experienced the altered state very deeply, I believe that the relaxation is the key to the success of my treatment."

2.

VALERIE JONES, aged 25 of Fallowfield, Manchester, also has multiple sclerosis and started to attend John Cain's healing sessions in May, 1978.

"When I saw my specialist in July, 1979," she says, "he thought I'd improved considerably and that I seemed to be coping well with my illness. He thinks that I'm having a remission from the condition."

Valerie has different views about this though and believes wholeheartedly that she has indeed received healing from John Cain. She explained why she is so certain on this score:

38

"It would seem that a victim of multiple sclerosis can go for long periods partially or wholly symptom-free.

Suddenly a symptom may reappear, remain for a long time then either go eventually or become steadily worse.

"In my case, symptoms do reappear, not for long periods, but just for odd days when I am capable of dispersing them by putting myself into 'the altered state' by concentrating my thoughts on John Cain or sometimes by looking at his photograph.

"I know my symptoms are there and I still have pain sometimes, but I can, through the altered state, overcome them. I feel I am in control of my illness rather than the other way round."

Valerie is convinced that she should by now have signs of wastage of the muscles but that has not happened.

It is an amazing sight to observe her in a healing session moving around with the grace and agility of sometimes a dancer and sometimes an athlete.

"When I first began to 'move' in the altered state," she recalls, "I was attending a physiotherapist who was helping me to relearn balance on one leg. During a healing session, I can quite easily balance on one shoulder, or my head! I can honestly say that I have never done exercises like this before I came to John Cain."

Valerie feels she has gained something from John Cain which because of the nature of her condition is very vital. She says: "Multiple scleroris is a soul-destroying condition. Remissions only bring temporary relief and depression is common. I have suffered no heavy depressions for a year now and find life more worth-while.

"But more important still is that I have changed permanently and can never imagine myself sinking so low again."

Valerie feels she owes more than just her improved physical health to Cain:

"He has given me back my sanity," she believes, "an interest in life and security and peace.

"I do not resent having contracted my present illness since without it I would never have met John Cain who has changed my life permanently for the better. I dread to think what things would be like now if I'd had to struggle on without him."

## 3

John Cain always knows just when or when not to interfere with patients' manipulations. The confidence with which he conducts his sessions is always backed up by the guidance he acknowledges comes from a higher intelligence. Cain asserts that they always know just how far to go and just how much healing a particular patient should receive. John Cain will only go to a patient during manipulation if he is directed to do so by the intelligence.

"Once," he relates, "I thought a patient was going to bang her head on an ornament; I put my hand under the head which stopped about two inches above my hand. The guides had made sure that there would be no injury."

It is a fact that there have never been any reported injuries after quite strenuous healing sessions. Some of the limb manipulations patients do whilst in the altered state compare well with the limbering up of athletes!

Why some patients lie down, passive, some move arms and legs rapidly, some stand on their heads, is not just chance. If a patient derives most benefit from a certain movement, no matter how bizarre that may appear to the observer, then he or she will probably continue that movement for the duration of the healing session.

MURIEL FOSTER, aged 65, from Hawthorn Road, Little Sutton, always sits upright when in the altered state. She has done so right from the first healing session she attended way back in 1975. If she lay down, she would not be able to twist her neck vigorously and thus her healing would not be so effective. When she came to John Cain, she was racked with pain from osteoarthritis. Her hands were mis-shapen, and her neck supported by an uncomfortable collar, worn day and night. One day, she felt certain she would be in a wheelchair, especially since the specialists she had consulted had told her there was nothing more they could do for her.

"I was very nervous on my first visit," she remembers, "but John Cain soon put me at my ease."

Muriel had a very good healing at this first session. She went into the altered state very quickly and began the manipulations to her neck, head, hands and legs which ensured that at the end of the session she could put the collar aside. She has never worn it since. She is also free from arthritic pain.

At the second healing session she attended, Muriel was surprised when John Cain identified deafness in her right ear; she had never mentioned it to him, being more concerned about her arthritis. Cain placed a clock to her right ear and said, 'when you go out of here you will hear'. She did and although the hearing in this ear is not one hundred per cent, she reports that it is considerably improved. Muriel has also been the subject of John Cain's irrepressible sense of humour.

Once, she was wearing lace-up shoes and had removed them for a healing session. When she tried to lace them up afterwards, she found that one hand was almost 'glued' to her knee. Cain told her to fasten her shoe with the other free hand. How she managed to tie a bow, she doesn't know, but she did though it took her ages as all the time she was trying to free her 'fixed' hand!

Muriel lost touch with John Cain when he moved from Eastham mainly because travelling over to Birkenhead was a long journey for her. However, in July, after a set-back in her health, a friend of hers, visiting Cain's, reported Muriel's condition to him.

Gout had been diagnosed and her left leg had swollen considerably. A week later after Cain had heard about Muriel he rang to ask her to come and speak to me about the book, also adding that he had been thinking of her all week.

Muriel told him that the swelling had gone down that very week, and it dawned on her suddenly that it must have been because Cain had been linking-up with her!

Muriel vowed that now she'd found John Cain again she wouldn't battle on her own any more and would continue to see him as often as she could.

4.

JILL FOSTER, from Hollin Lane, Whitchurch, Salop had suffered with a rare disease, sarcoidosis, since she was about eighteen years of age. It is a vicious condition, affecting the lungs and thus the breathing and causes the skin to become red and puffy.

It had affected Jill's face more than any other part of her body but she also had unsightly red lumps all over her arms and legs. She could not do anything, even walk upstairs, without becoming very breathless.

Apart from suffering greatly from the physical effects of this disease, Jill was affected psychologically to a terrible degree. "I was continually depressed," she recalled. "I had no confidence in myself and very little energy. In fact, I spent most of the time in bed.

"A Harley Street specialist could only suggest drugs which treated the symptoms of the disease but not the cause."

Jill had been told when she first contracted the disease that there was no cure but that it might possibly 'burn itself out'.

However, she was so desperately unhappy that when she heard of John Cain through a relative, she decided that she had nothing to lose by going to see him.

During her first visit in January, 1975, John Cain put Jill into the 'altered state' simply by putting his hands near her head. "I had no previous knowledge of Cain's method of healing. He didn't speak to me and I just floated into a reclining position. My husband watched me during the whole of the session and remarked that I didn't move so much as a finger for nearly three hours; I thought I'd only been 'out' for ten minutes!

"During the healing I felt an intense heat emanating from John Cain's hands. At the end of the session I felt a tremendous spiritual upliftment and my depression disappeared temporarily."

Similar sessions followed as Jill visited John Cain each week and she began to feel better all round. Her confidence returned, her depression became more spasmodic and she discovered new-found energy. Her breathing also improved and although there was as yet no obvious improvement in her physical condition the change in her mental outlook enabled her to cope with her condition. She realised later that this change had to precede her physical healing.

A few months after beginning sessions at Cain's, Jill began to do Yoga exercises whilst in the altered state.

"I was most surprised to find myself tumbling about John Cain's room," she says, "and found I had no control over these exercises, never knowing in advance what I would do."

Jill has thought about these phenomena many times and has concluded that whilst in the altered state patients have access to a universal knowledge which goes back centuries and therefore often know instinctively what to do.

"I had no knowledge at all of Yoga and would like to make that quite clear," she says. "I found out later that every exercise I did was

42

an authentic Yoga movement and related to an organ or part of my body which had been affected by the condition."

Jill continued the exercises at home and eventually found that she could do this by simply lying on the floor and doing whatever she felt impelled to do. Gradually she noticed some improvement in her physical condition.

Her hopes soared as with time her improvement became more noticeable and she cut down on the drugs she had been taking.

Two years ago Jill and her husband became helpers at Cain's public sessions and looking back, Jill feels that this was the turning-point in her recovery and her improvement accelerated from then on.

"I can honestly say that I am ninety-nine per cent better. I no longer take drugs, I feel fitter than I have done for years and my skin has almost completely recovered from the terrible effects of the disease. My energy most days is limitless. I owe my life to John Cain."

Jill is well aware that the medical profession could turn round and say that her disease has 'burned itself out', but the extra years of happiness she has been given would not have been hers if she had waited for that to happen.

"In any case," she says, "I have no confidence in that prognosis at all because a woman who was in hospital with me when I first had the disease still has it very badly."

5.

It took doctors three years to diagnose the condition of SHEILA DODD, aged 32 of Wilkinson Street, Ellesmere Port.

On the surface she looked all right but she was in terrible pain all over and found walking very difficult.

She says: "Various doctors I saw just looked at me as if I were stupid when I tried to explain my symptoms."

Sheila became practically bed-bound and her husband took much time from work to look after her and their young child, then aged two. Then a colleague of Dave Dodd, Sheila's husband, mentioned John Cain to him. Dave's first reaction was very sceptical, he remembers.

Then he thought, 'well, we've tried everything else, so why not?'

Once the name John Cain has entered a person's life, it often keeps reappearing, as many a person told me, whilst researching for this book.

Dave Dodd now kept seeing Cain's name everywhere and he felt a strong motivation to take Sheila to him.

But it took him nearly six months to persuade her to go. As she says: "I'd been so disillusioned by the medical profession, that I'd given up. Nobody had taken any notice of me and I thought why should John Cain?"

Dave describes their first visit to Bromborough in 1977. "Immediately we both felt there was something special about the atmosphere. Sheila lay down on a mattress and went into a light relaxed state. Nothing spectacular happened but as we drove home she said how much better she felt psychologically."

After a few more healing sessions, Sheila proved to be very receptive and went into an altered state very easily.

Although Sheila still did not know what name to give to her condition, John Cain said that he thought she had inflammation in her back.

Sheila became very ill, so ill in fact that she had almost trebled the dose of pain-killing tablets prescribed for her. This was a dangerous act, but in desperation, she had been unaware of how many tablets she was taking.

She was taken to hospital and after many tests, came the verdict: Ankylosing Spondilitis, an acute rheumatic inflammation of the spine. The outlook was bleak. In ten to fifteen years, Sheila could expect to be permanently bent as her bones fused together.

Even though she had not yet received physical healing from Cain, Sheila still felt compelled to see him.

"There were times," she told me, "when I had to drag myself there."

There now followed an interesting change in Sheila during the healing sessions.

Previously she had always lain quietly but suddenly one night she began to self-manipulate with an agility that astonished her husband who knew how limited her mobility was.

After a few months the pain lessened all over and she began to pick up the threads again of a normal life.

"Now her condition seems stabilized," reports a jubilant husband. "We like to keep in contact with Cain because we think it is important for my wife's continuing progress. We had a telephone

44

installed especially so that we could ring Cain if ever she has a flare-up.

"Once, at the height of a particularly bad flare-up, I rang John and though it was very late he said not to worry. He told me to move my hands over her painful areas and he would link-up with us. Her pain went in a very short time!"

Now, Sheila feels that her future is brighter and thinks that what Cain has done for her is 'fantastic'.

Her husband believes that as wonderful as the physical healing has been, the spiritual help given to his wife by John Cain has been very therapeutic.

"Cain has enabled us both to live a happier and fuller life and we can never thank him enough."

## 6.

When JOAN KELLY, aged 67, from Bromborough, came to John Cain's in 1975, she had had arthritis for fourteen years. She was so bad that she couldn't sit, stand or lie down in any comfort. In fact, she just didn't know what to do with herself!

The first time she came to John Cain's, she went into a beautiful relaxed state:

"I remember thinking when Cain put his hands under my back and lifted me up slightly that I could have died just at that moment; it was so peaceful."

She did not die, however. Far from it! She is now able to get round with great mobility and comes twice weekly still to John Cain's because she feels the contact with him has helped her to get over the death of her husband, Bill. She also gets great relief from a hiatus hernia which she has been told may not respond satisfactorily to an operation.

She is also grateful for the help which John Cain gave to her husband who had had major surgery for cancer.

"He came into the hospital to visit him and his wound healed much faster than the surgeon expected and he was surprised. When they sent him home, I knew he would probably die but John Cain still came to give him healing and right up to the end he was in good spirits and did not need heavy pain-killing injections until three days before he died. I never expected a cure but there is no doubt that John Cain helped him bear his condition with strength."


7.


MONA JONES, of Bickerton Avenue, Bebington, aged 74 years, was decorating when I spoke to her.

"I couldn't have done this two years ago!" she said with feeling.

That was before she went to see John Cain in Autumn 1977. Mona had just recovered from a nervous breakdown but in addition she had two long-standing physical complaints which constantly 'dragged her down'.

"I was just amazed," she says, "at what I saw at Bromborough that first visit and when a bed became empty I lay down. I never even met John Cain that night and yet I still came away feeling marvellous."

Patients may attend sessions for weeks before they actually have personal contact with Cain. To some, this presents a psychological barrier and they feel they are not receiving any 'proper' help. But Mona Jones' story gives the lie to this theory because it was weeks before she spoke to Cain.

The fact that people often ask for John Cain to be pointed out to them demonstrates how informal the sessions are and how little he is interested in projecting himself by fancy introductions or ostentatious actions. He does not need to; his patients do that for him when they talk about what he has done for them.

Mona Jones describes her first visit:

"I went into the 'altered state'as soon as a lady helper placed her hands on my head and eyes. I felt an intense heat from her hands and I didn't want to move or get up for ages.

"When I did 'come to', I felt on top of the world! I went home and slept like a log!"

Mona began to make regular trips to Cain's sessions and when she eventually spoke to him, told him of her breakdown. Cain said to her: "You will have no more breakdowns; you can be sure of that."

Mona also told him about the colitis she had had and the surgical belt worn for back trouble for twenty-nine years.

After only a few sessions she says that she no longer needed the belt and has never worn it since. Her colitis condition is also stabilised.

She has this to say about John Cain:

"He has made a new woman of me and I'm eternally grateful to him."


## 8.


DOROTHY BLACKWELL, aged 54 from Kirkby, will never forget the day in June, 1977 when she sneezed violently!

Up until that day, she had been recovering quite nicely from a spinal fusion operation, and now, just two months after that operation, before the bones had set, she had sneezed with such force and upset everything. Now, she could not walk, was in the most terrible pain and could not sit down at all.

"We can't do any more for you," the hospital staff told her, "as far as we're concerned the graft has taken. Maybe in six months or so you'll sit down again properly."

But Dorothy could not. The pain was so intense. Life now was seen from a lying position; even a drive in the car was on a special mattress which replaced the front passenger seat. She had acupuncture without success then returned to hospital because she hoped they could help her.

Although Andy Blackwell is very sceptical about healers and the like, he nevertheless felt so desperate for his wife's condition that he cut out a newspaper article about John Cain and took it into hospital for Dot to see.

"I didn't believe," said Andy, "but I didn't say so to my wife. And when she came out of hospital in July 1978 and was bed-ridden, she said she would like to go to Bromborough. I knew she wouldn't be able to make it, so I offered to go one Wednesday night by myself just to see what went on."

That was on the Wednesday morning. Andy went off to work, and when he returned, to his surprise Dot was up and ready to go. She had arranged for their daughter to help her and accompany her to the Civic Hall, that evening.

After a great struggle Andy took Dot into the hall. What happened next he remembers very clearly:

"John Cain came up to Dot and *sat* her in a chair; he then laid his hands on her head and she immediately went into some form of

47

trance or deep sleep. I turned my head away to hide my tears because she looked so peaceful after being in pain for such a long time. She was 'out' for about half-an-hour and during that time moved her hands to the music as though playing the piano.

"John Cain had told Dot to look at his photograph the next day at 7 p.m.

"The next day, at that time, the 'phone rang and I answered it. It was for Dot and I turned to tell her but found she had gone 'out' again. I was so worried I sat on the bed and watched her. When she came round she said she had heard me call but could not open her eyes. From then we have visited John Cain three to four times a week. The relief from pain has been unbelievable. A very strange thing was that at John Cain's, Dot could sit for several hours but when she got home, she couldn't. This continued for three months until one week-end, Dot just said, "I'm going to sit in the car." She did and since May 1979 she has been leading a normal life.

"But she keeps going to John Cain's because with every visit she feels stronger. I myself could never repay John Cain for the joy he has given me and my family by restoring my wife to health."

It is a sad fact that where a specialist or consultant has been told of the work of John Cain and has agreed that he is indeed doing good, because of the stringent attitude of the B.M.A., these medics cannot speak out for him. In Dot's case, the acupuncturist consultant is fully aware of John Cain's work and when he asked Dot whom did she think was doing her the most good, himself or John Cain, Dot said without hesitation, "Oh, John Cain." "Well," the consultant remarked, "come in about three months to me."

But despite the tight-lipped attitude of the medical profession, John Cain's name is spreading and this is borne out by this little story Andy Blackwell tells.

"After leaving one of John Cain's special healing sessions on a Sunday morning, at about 1.30 a.m., I was driving though the Mersey Tunnel with Dot lying in the back, covered over with a blanket. A Tunnel police car followed me and stopped me before leaving. I had swerved slightly on to the metal studs, the police told me. 'But I'm not drunk,' I said, 'I've been to see John Cain with my wife'."

The policeman's instant reaction amazed Andy.

"O.K. Mate, carry on."

"This man," says Andy, "gets you out of trouble when he's not with you!"

## 9

BARBARA HICKS, aged 50, from Alistair Drive, Bromborough had a stroke in 1973. She was only 42. The stroke left her completely paralysed down the right side and her right hand was immobilised with the fingers locked in the palm. Her specialist told her husband that she would never speak again.

Apart from being completely dependent on her husband to do the housework, cook and dress her, Barbara suffered greatly from her inability to communicate. Her speech therapist had worked with her for eighteen months and eventually discharged her, saying she had done all she could; it was all up to Barbara from now on.

In 1977, feeling very depressed about her future, Barbara was taken to a public healing session at Bromborough.

"I was very doubtful about the help I might receive," she told me. "But John Cain really opened the door of life to me. I found great peace and felt at one with the world whilst in the altered state."

Physically there was very little change over the next few months, but Barbara found that mentally she became very relaxed.

Then after about four or five months something started to happen. She suddenly began to move her right arm and leg whilst in the altered state.

"From that time," she recalls, "my improvement was quite rapid. Now I am able to walk better, faster and further without tiring. I am no longer depressed and I can use my right hand to cut up food. I no longer dread the ring of the telephone if I am in the house alone and answer it without fear."

Each time Barbara visits her specialist he is surprised at how well she looks and keeps asking her if she is breathless or has headaches. The symptoms he expects her to have just aren't there!

To crown it all, Barbara used to have two heart murmurs, but on her last medical examination in June 1979, only one could be found! Alfred Hicks, Barbara's husband, is very puzzled about the healing she received from John Cain but accepts that it has happened.

"All I know," he says "is that since Barbara went to John Cain, physically and mentally she has shown a marked improvement. She is doing all her own work in the house now and is not dependent on me to any great degree at all.

"I don't pretend to understand anything at all about this type of healing. I am not particularly religious and can't see it therefore as an act of God. But I think John Cain definitely possesses a great gift."

## 10.

It is often the wife or husband of a sick person who will make the arrangements to visit John Cain. Driven by desperation that nothing else can be done medically and the fact they themselves are suffering from lack of sleep and stress that an illness so often brings to a household, they take courage in both hands. They often know they will have to fight scepticism.

BETTY CHARLES, from Maghull, is never sorry she looked up Cain's telephone number after reading about him in a local newspaper. This was in 1977. Her husband, Ron, had had arthritis since 1966 and by now it had attacked most joints. The various drugs he had tried had not helped at all to control its progress.

He had kept up his job as a sales representative by sheer determination to keep going but he was having to walk with the aid of two sticks. Just how long he could keep up with his job often worried him.

They arrived at Bromborough Civic Hall to find it packed and had to wait quite some time before Ron had his healing.

Betty relates that Ron didn't feel anything very much at this first session and it was only really to please her that he agreed to come a second time.

At this second session, things were quite different.

John Cain came to Ron where he sat on a chair and put his hands on his neck and shoulders. Ron remembers what happened:

"I felt terrific heat from Cain's hands as he manipulated my neck. Cain warned me that I might experience severe pain but that my neck would improve.

"That night I was troubled by acute pains but by the morning the pain in my neck had gone and it has never returned."

Ron Charles continued to visit the Hall two or three times a week and after a few weeks did not need his sticks.

Although he still suffers with arthritis he is so much better and derives much benefit from the continued healing.

Betty Charles also suffered from headaches and soon found that after she started receiving healing from John Cain, her pain went and she slept better. Almost from the very beginning, she has been able to go into a very deep sleep whilst in the altered state.

"I am often unaware of the music being played so that is how I know how deeply I have relaxed."

* * * * *

John Cain is the last person to claim that he is always able to heal instantly.

He does not delve into the reasons why some people are healed outright, whilst others become progressively better.

Two people, both with the same condition may respond differently to the healing; the one receiving almost instant help, the other perhaps not receiving any noticeable help for weeks. Nearly always, though, from my observations and interviews, I discovered that some benefit had eventually been received from the contact with Cain, be it physical or spiritual.

Cain prefers to accept everything as it happens and leaves the fathoming to others. However, he is confident enough to state that ninety-five per cent of cases respond in some way.

What cannot be denied is that outright healings by Cain are not rare occurrences and they just cannot be dismissed lightly.

* * * * *

11.

IVY GIBSON, aged 68 from Little Sutton, Merseyside, went into John Cain's centre almost bent up double and hardly able to walk. When she came out she did a dance!

51

As fantastic as that story sounds, she assures me that this was just how it happened. In fact when she went to visit the girls with whom she worked they couldn't believe it when she danced in front of them also.

This was in 1975. She had been told to learn to live with a slipped disc and arthritis of the hip and was in agony most of the time, with only slight relief from pain killers.

She remembers that first healing session well:

"I went into an altered state straight away and after a short time, was aware that my legs were moving with great agility. This surprised me because I knew I could not move normally like this. There was no pain at all which also amazed me. Afterwards, I realised that I had had a really marvellous healing. I continued to visit Cain every week and grew stronger all the time. I don't understand how it happened but I now take no tablets and have no more pain and that's good enough for me." Ivy also received healing from John Cain for haemorrhages behind her eyes.

"They told me at the eye hospital," says Ivy, "that I would never see properly again with my right eye and that the left one would soon be affected in the same way.

"Well, after healing from John Cain I can still see fine with my left eye and in fact my right eye has improved."

In August, 1978, Ivy hurt her back again. She was told to lie on her back for three weeks and not attempt to get up.

Her husband soon did something about that. He rang John Cain and he agreed to make a home visit for which Ivy is eternally grateful, because she knows how precious little time he has to make house calls.

"John Cain came into my room and put me in the altered state," Ivy remembers, "and after only eight minutes, I stood on the floor, pain-free!

"I went back to bed to rest but the next day got up as normal and I've never had any more back trouble since!"

## 12

MABEL DAVIES, aged 60, of Millersdale Close, Eastham received an outright healing from John Cain in the Spring of 1977.

For thirteen years prior to this time, she was crippled with osteo-arthritis. Her condition had started when she lost the use of the fingers in her right hand and right arm. A visit to the doctor's resulted in a prescription for pain-killers.

But the condition worsened. It spread to her neck, back and left arm. A specialist was consulted and Mabel underwent numerous tests which confirmed her condition.

She was by now unable to lift her arms, comb her hair, clean her teeth, and her muscles began to waste.

She was given traction and a surgical collar to wear but neither helped her complaint. Black-outs and impaired eyesight now caused her a lot of trouble and the prognosis was that in time she might not be able to move at all.

Mabel enquired about specially-designed knives and forks to help with eating because she could no longer grip and her hands had become mis-shapen, but as it turned out she was not going to need these aids.

Looking through a local newspaper in 1977, she read an article about John Cain and the help he was giving to arthritics like herself.

"I decided to go and see him," Mabel recalls.

"I had no idea what sort of man he would be. But as I sat talking to him about my problem, I felt very relaxed and at ease with him. John Cain did not make any rash promises. He just said, 'We will see what we can do.'

"To begin with, I was told to take my coat off. John Cain told me to sit down on the couch whilst he knelt at my side. He put his hand above my head and told me not to stop my neck or hands from moving if this happened. The heat from his hand was intense. I felt marvellous and so relaxed. It was altogether a wonderful experience. I felt myself being drawn back into a lying position and yet John Cain was not touching me at all."

Mabel Davies felt now what can only be described as electric shocks throughout her body. Her neck started to move and she felt her bones being manipulated. She described being aware of every-thing and yet unaware at the same time and could not open her eyes, a description of most people's experience when in 'the altered state'.

When she eventually sat up, John Cain was just standing looking at her.

"I remember then that he asked me to turn my head and look behind, to the right and then to the left, which I did. He handed me my coat which I swung around my shoulders which was something wonderful to me. John Cain just smiled at me and handed me a cup which I held with my thumb and forefinger, something I hadn't done for years. I knew then that I had had a spontaneous healing and was overwhelmed by the experience.

"There was no talk about money. John Cain's greatest reward is just seeing a patient walk out through the door, healed. And I was one of those patients."

Mabel describes her walk home as that of someone re-born. She felt so excited she wanted to skip! Her own daughter, recognising her coat as she passed her window, could not believe it was her mother and had to run out and call after her.

"She couldn't believe her eyes," says Mabel. " 'Mum, what's happened!' she cried out, and I flung my arms into the air and behind my back. She laughed and cried at the same time. After thirteen years I was a normal, healthy person again."

Mabel never forgot the healing she received at John's hands and continued to attend his sessions, finding great comfort from them.

In 1978, Mabel lost her youngest son. It was a great loss to her. She prayed hard the night before his funeral, for strength; she couldn't bear the thought of going through the service.

A strange thing happened at the church.

"During the service," she relates, "I suddenly felt limp and my eyes closed. I was aware of what was going on around me but I just seemed to be floating. I must have been escorted out of the church and put to bed because I don't remember anything else until I awoke in bed hours later, smiling, with no tears. My daughter was there and she explained. John Cain had been at the back of the church. He told me later that he had received a message that there was something I did not want to witness. So he had been there to help. My prayer had been answered because I did not see my son taken away from me."

Mabel feels that at the session, whilst in 'the altered state', she has her son handed her back to her as a baby, because to her, as her youngest child, he is still her baby.

54

"This makes it easier for me to bear his tragic death and lifts the depression which some days crowds in on me."

\* \* \* \* \*

## 13.

The large public healing demonstration John Cain conducted at the Philharmonic Hall, Liverpool on September 9th, 1977, was the first high spot in his career as a healer.

Before the packed audience, he put on a remarkable demonstration of his healing gift.

Cain did not do anything different that night; he did not suddenly turn into a 'platform' healer and introduce himself or his healing with fancy words. He allowed other, more articulate people to introduce him. Cain merely put into practice what he preaches and healed.

In the days following the demonstration, Cain received well over a hundred telephone calls testifying either to instant healing or relief of some kind received on that night.

One of the instant healings that actually took place on the platform and was seen by hundreds is related by a very grateful, HELEN KILLEN, aged 58, from Bootle, Liverpool.

She had suffered from cervical spondilitis for over twenty-five years and that night, she had come to the Philharmonic Hall wearing a very heavy support neck-collar.

She had never been free from pain in all those years and her medical record would fill several pages. Suffice it to say that she had, over the years, endured traction; injections, manipulation under anaesthetic; heat treatment; drugs of all kinds, one addictive; hospital treatment – all to little avail.

Helen believes her healing began the night before she attended the public demonstration:

She says, "I was in terrible pain and looked forward to the next night with great hope. I had seen a photograph of John Cain and went into a deep sleep with his face in my mind."

The next day she recalls being very hot all over, when usually she was so cold and experienced an itching in her back which she could not explain.

Another strange event took place which Helen also sees as being linked with her healing.

"My brother arrived unexpectedly from the South of England," she told me, "and gave us a lift into Liverpool. Consequently, we were too early for the public demonstration and went into a hotel close to the hall for a drink and to pass some time.

"I recognised John Cain, who was also in the hotel, and to my own surprise and without hesitation, I went up to him and asked him would he have a 'go' at my neck. He asked me how long I'd worn the collar and then he said, 'right, you're the one I want when I ask people to come up.' Later, when Cain asked people to raise their hands if they wanted healing on the platform, my friend had to support my arm because I was in too much pain to lift it myself."

Evenutally, Helen got to the platform and John Cain came to her. Helen described what happened next:

"Cain unfastened my collar and I cringed. I relaxed though as he spoke quietly and then he began to twist my neck from side to side and then around. He put my chin forward on to my chest and bent my head backwards. My mother, watching in the audience, told me afterwards that she was in agony for me because she knew I could not normally do such movements. There were other people in that hall also who knew that I could never move in this way."

Helen recalls that after the healing on the platform, she felt uplifted and completely free from pain.

"I have never looked back from that night," she says jubilantly. "It used to take me hours to get ready, now I'm up at seven-thirty, do my housework and shopping and run a small business without any trouble at all.

"I cannot say I no longer have the condition called spondilitis, but the pain is an awful long time in coming back!

"I take no tablets and the lack of drugs alone is surely something not to be ignored. My system now has time to heal completely."

Helen Killen sums up what John Cain means to her as someone with a quite strong religious faith:

"I don't know what John Cain has but think he must be being used by God or the Holy Spirit to heal. In answer to the criticism of him by people from within my own religion and any other religion, I say that what happened to me has only strengthened my faith.

56

"When I see John Cain at work, I see an ordinary man working hard and leaving himself open to ridicule. In the face of that, he just carries on and relieves suffering every day of his life. That is all that matters."

Helen hits out at those critics who call Cain's method of healing 'mass hypnosis' or 'mind-over-matter'.

"If I thought I could have cured myself by being 'hypnotised' or by just thinking I had no pain, I would have done it years ago!" she says. "I refuse to believe, however, that 'auto-suggestion' could remove harmful calcium deposits lodged for years in joints."


## 14.


The instant healing RENE CRIMES received from John Cain in February, 1978, came as quite a surprise to her.

Rene, aged 44, from Whitby, Ellesmere Port, was merely sitting talking to John Cain about the possibility of a private healing for her arthritic hands and feet.

"John Cain said he didn't do private healings," explained Rene, "and we were just sitting having a cup of tea.

"He went out of the room for a moment and when he returned he placed what seemed like white cards on each of my hands. Immediately I experienced a 'pins and needles' sensation in my hands. Mr Cain told me not to fight any other feelings I might have and then I must have gone to 'sleep' because I don't remember any more."

Rene's husband, Jim, carries on the story:

"Cain sat on the opposite side of the room and at no time did he come near my wife. He just moved each of his hands in turn and my wife, in a very heavy sleep, imitated his movements with her own hands. Cain did the same with his feet and Rene copied him.

"I just sat amazed at what I saw and couldn't believe that it was happening to us."

Afterwards, Rene remembers that she could move her hands and feet without pain for the first time in two years. She stood on her toes on Cain's instructions which was an impossible movement to her before her healing. Previously also she had been unable to hold a kettle or an iron and now she could clench her fist easily. The 'white cards' turned out to be Cain's photographs, back-to-front, and this was all Cain had used to accomplish this remarkable instant healing!

Amazing as it sounds, Rene received instant healing for another condition that very same afternoon.

"I no longer needed to take drugs for the epileptic fits I'd been having quite frequently before coming to Cain. My doctor's reaction when I told him I had stopped having these fits was to make out another prescription and to tell me to 'keep taking the tablets'! I'm grateful to say that I have not had another fit since visiting Cain and do not need drugs of any kind."

Rene and Jim Crimes both say their lives have changed dramatically since knowing Cain.

"We now come to help John Cain with his healing," say Rene, "and my husband who was once a darts champion, gave away all his trophies and has given up the game completely to devote more of his time to Cain."

15.

MARY PRICE, aged 54, from Neath in South Wales, had been practically bed-ridden for ten years with osteoarthritis. She was also very troubled with bowel disorder, stomach ulcers and had a breathing problem.

"I was in such a bad way," Mary recalls, "that I even planned my own funeral!"

Her son-in-law read the article about Cain in *The Weekly News* in July, 1979 and wrote off to Cain for more information.

Mary is convinced that her healing began from the minute she read Cain's reply which was in the form of the usual letter sent in answer to enquiries about his healing.

One particular sentence in that letter had great significance for Mary: 'The first signs of the healing are often experienced with more vitality and a brighter outlook, better sleep and a sense of inner upliftment as the healing forces begin to bring about easement.'

She reports, after reading the letter that she did indeed feel 'uplifted' and cried with relief. Then to the astonishment of her family, she asked to be dressed in outdoor clothes and requested to be taken to a new store she'd heard so much about. This was quite unlike her usual behaviour as she had made very few outside trips and spent most of her time dressed in a nightdress.

The following day she surprised them all again when she endorsed a suggestion that her son-in-law had made previously that they should invest in a caravan. The reason for this was soon to be made quite clear.

Mary now felt she just had to visit Cain.

"Something was driving me," she says.

And so on the 10th August they made the long journey up from South Wales to Cain's centre in Birkenhead.

Mary was wheeled into his centre in her wheelchair and was assisted on to a couch.

"I lay down," reports Mary, "and when Cain came to me I felt terrific heat from his hands. My back was stretched without any contact from Cain and I felt totally at peace for about three hours! I had no pain at all."

Mary walked out of Cain's centre and startled her husband, Evan. "I thought it was just fantastic," he says.

Needless to say, on the long journey to Wales, Mary was very excited and did not stop talking about her remarkable healing.

She reports that her friends in Wales were astonished by her recovers.

Two weeks later, Mary felt she needed the contact with Cain to be strengthened. She had been so ill for such a long time that her confidence in her recovery needed to be reinforced. Now, that caravan she'd been so keen about came in handy. They could afford to come up and stay near Cain for a week at very little expense.

At the centre, during that week in August, 1979, her healing was strengthened and she reports that she experienced stronger self-manipulations each time. When I saw her on August 26th, she told me how marvellous she felt and certainly she looked it. She was no longer taking pain-killers for arthritis as her pain had gone. She also told me with much pleasure that her wheelchair, which had developed a puncture on the day she received her first healing, had never been out of the boot of the car!

Mary was delighted to be able to say also that her other conditions had improved greatly also.

Kay Phillips, aged 31, also from South Wales and Mary's daughter also received an instant healing for deafness in her right ear. This she had had since she was eighteen months old! Mary's husband also, reported that a worsening deafness in both of his ears had been halted by Cain and was able to add that his hearing had actually improved.

Certainly the Prices will never regret investing in that caravan which enabled them to have a healing holiday!


## 16.


Washing nappies is nobody's dream of a pleasant occupation, but to SHEILA SPEIRS, aged 49, from Cranleigh Road, Woolton, Liverpool, washing her grandson's is nothing short of a miracle. For twenty-five years she had endured 'crucifying' pain and various gynaecological operations, internal haemorrhages and thrombosis and arthritis in her knees and neck. The pain, in her own words 'had beaten me'.

By November, 1976, she faced up to one major fact; there was nothing that orthodox medicine could do to help her; one last try to conquer the pain was a spinal injection which could be repeated every three months, if successful. This failed, in fact, made her vomit, and she knew then there was no further hope.

The name John Cain kept cropping up in conversation with Sheila and her friends. But like many other people before, she heard it, then put it from her mind. In any case, she was so drugged half the time and in such pain, that normal straight thinking out of problems or taking any action never occurred to her.

Then Sheila went for her final injection at Walton Hospital. She was so ill after it that her daughter, unable to see her for a fortnight because of a bus-strike, was horrified at her deterioration when next she saw her. The hospital had made their final pronouncement, 'there is no more we can do'. Sheila remembers their kindness to this day. Her husband, Douglas, had been told by their doctor, and unknown to Sheila, that she had at the most, twelve months left.

On October 7th, 1977, Sheila's sister offered to accompany her to the Bromborough Civic Hall. Sheila's story from then on, is best told by herself:

"At Bromborough, my sister had a terrible time getting me into the hall; I could only walk bent over practically in two so Maureen was taking all my weight. We sat and waited for this man, John Cain. Everyone seemed to be so serene and I thought, 'If they're sick, then I'm Charles Atlas!' I said in no uncertain terms that they'd never get

60

me down on a mattress.

"Time passed and I grew agitated with the pain. I'd expected to be seen first but here I was just waiting. The pain was really getting at me and angry now, I muttered to my sister, 'let's go.' We had been there about forty minutes and I was annoyed because I felt cheated that these people getting treatment didn't look sick or in pain. Suddenly, I couldn't take any more. 'Let's get out of here and let me scream my head off,' I said to Maureen.

"I was really embarrassed as I tried to get out of the hall and not fall over people lying down. Maureen was practically carrying me out to the foyer when a voice said, 'give her a drink of water.' Someone sat me on a chair by a table and I took a sip of water. I discovered after that this person was Audrey Cain.

"John Cain then came to me and asked me, 'where is the pain?'

"I was in such a state," recalls Sheila, "that I was rude to him and told him to leave me alone."

But John Cain, quietly persistent, asked Sheila to close her eyes.

She continued her story:

"Then he placed one hand on my lower left side and the other on the lower part of my back at the base of my spine.

"Instantly it felt as if a finger was gently entering into my spine on the left hand side of the spine and pressing. Immediately, the whole diabolical pain throughout my body went. It could not have been more than sixty seconds when I said, 'You have got it. It has gone.' It felt as if someone had pressed a light switch off and the pain went as quickly as the light would.

"I looked at John Cain and said to him, 'Mate, you have had one great miracle tonight. You don't know the half of it.' By that I meant that he just didn't know what a fantastic healing I had had. I felt as if I wanted to put up a plaque there and then on that hall wall to testify to his great healing."

After her instant healing, which indeed can only be described as miraculous, Sheila Speirs got in and out of her sister's car without any trouble. At her sister's home, Sheila wanted to open the garage doors and did so; her sister's friend suffered shock when she saw Sheila and her niece, who was fifteen at the time, was amazed when she walked up the stairs unaided.

Sheila returned to Bromborough the next week and chose a seat furthest away from the stage. She tried to be inconspicuous because her instant healing the week previous had caused quite a stir among the regular helpers and patients.

61

She felt humbled at the fact she had received such a 'miraculous cure' and yet some of these patients who had been coming for a long time and receiving a more progressive healing, which is often the case, were so overjoyed at her instant healing.

Sheila Speirs and her husband, Douglas Speirs, both swear that they will never forget what John Cain has done for them. Every day of their life they do something to publicise his name and spread the word about him.

Sheila also pays tribute to Audrey Cain:

"She is completely dedicated and I think is his anchor."

"John Cain is no saint, but he has a God-given gift and he is a truly dedicated healer; he never gets tired of tending sick people. I have never seen an expression of boredom in his face."

Sheila, in her publicity campaign, admits that it is hard for friends to believe she has been healed and says that some didn't admit she had been until about twelve months later. Then they said, "Yes, Sheila, we do believe it is a miracle now."

And what of the reaction to Sheila Speirs' fantastic recovery by her own family doctor?

It is a sad reflection on the limitations placed on doctors that they cannot openly come out and say, "well, this patient was certainly very ill; there was nothing more I or the specialist could do; drugs alleviated her pain but she was in one awful state. She has been made well again by a healer, and the most important thing is that she *is* well.'

That kind of statement will only be possible when the medical profession begins to look more closely at unorthodox medicine.

From my research, the usual comments range from 'rubbish', 'baloney', 'impossible', and one even said, because the patient had stopped taking some tablets after Cain had healed her, 'you'll be sorry!'

Where has the compassion gone from a profession which is after all primarily concerned with healing?

In Sheila's case, there was certainly disbelief at first.

Her doctor's reaction though, after the news had sunk in that she was indeed perfectly well, was that he did believe whole-heartedly there are gifted people like Cain.

Douglas Speirs reports that the doctor still checks up now and again to ask if she has maintained her healing, not because he wants to gloat if she has had a set-back, but because he is genuinely pleased for her recovery.

Sheila has not been slow in getting in touch with the British Medical Association but, she says, they have 'tactfully avoided my suggestion that they openly admit to the cures of this man who is truly a servant of God, yet who still remains humble and dedicated to helping those in despair.'

It is her great hope that one day, the medical profession will work hand-in-hand with men like John Cain.

\* \* \*

Sometimes when a member of a family is healed, there are repercussions on other members in the form of 'strange' phenomena.

In the case of Sheila Speirs, an extraordinary happening took place miles away, in Grassau, West Germany, at the time of her 'instant' healing.

Douglas Speirs, Sheila's husband, remembers every detail of this strange incident:

"On Friday night, the 7th October, 1977, my daughter, who was working in a hotel in Germany, was struck down with a mysterious illness. She was taken violently ill with pain in her head, back and side, and vomited so badly that a doctor had to be sent for. He prescribed various medicines for her fever and pain and she stayed that way for six days. She had no sleep at all and was sick daily.

"The night she was taken ill was the very same night and the exact hour my wife received her marvellous healing from John Cain."

Douglas posted a photograph of John Cain to her which she placed under her pillow. That night she slept for the first time since her illness and awoke the next morning refreshed and completely cured.

17.

Douglas Speirs' gratitude to John Cain resulted in him broadcasting a personal testimony about his wife's marvellous recovery on Radio Merseyside in 1978. Many people heard it and it was relayed at least five times during one day.

It was a lucky day for JEAN SWIFT, aged 50, of 23, Howbeck Close, Birkenhead. She heard the broadcast and remembered also that she had seen an article in *The News of the World*.

The name John Cain stayed in her mind.

After fourteen years of pain resulting from disc degeneration, a history of high blood pressure, sleeplessness and headaches, she was in pretty poor shape. Pain-killers gave her temporary relief only.

In June of 1978, she decided to attend a public healing session at Bromborough. She was so apprehensive she just observed and would not lie down.

Something made her go a second time and this time she took courage in both hands and lay down. She remembers bright lights, though her eyes were shut, and a feeling of heaviness in her eyelids. There was no noticeable change in her physical condition, however.

For some people, this is enough to convince them that John Cain cannot help them, and they do not return. Always he tries to convey the message that people must not expect miracles and although many are sensible about this, there are those who expect too much all at once.

Jean Swift is very glad she had enough sense to return because gradually, after only a few more sessions, her headaches and back improved until suddenly one day, she realised that she was no longer in pain.

Jean Swift has become one of John Cain's helpers now and says: "This gives me the greatest satisfaction. And it is wonderful to be able to help John Cain in return for the help he has given me."

Jean's husband, Ken, has also received great relief from violent headaches which caused him to be very depressed. He, too, is a dedicated helper now.

18.

ROBERT OWEN, aged 47 from Blakeley, Manchester, considered that his own pain and loss of sleep was a nuisance but that his wife's arthritic condition was in more need of healing than his own.

So when he read an article about John Cain in July 1979 in the 'Weekly News', he immediately thought of bringing her.

Robert decided to have healing for himself on their second visit to Cain. He remembers clearly what happened:

64

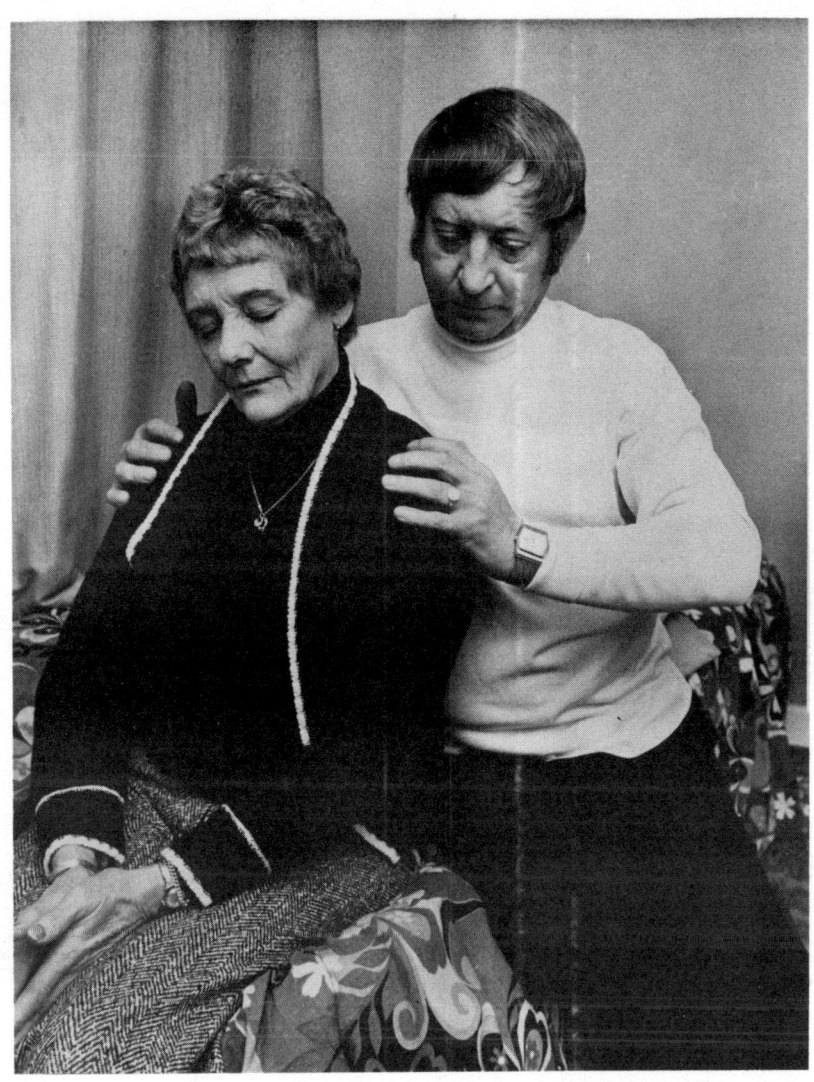

*This arthritic patient, who also suffered severe pain, was immediately relaxed. Her case of a spontaneous relief from pain caused considerable comment.*

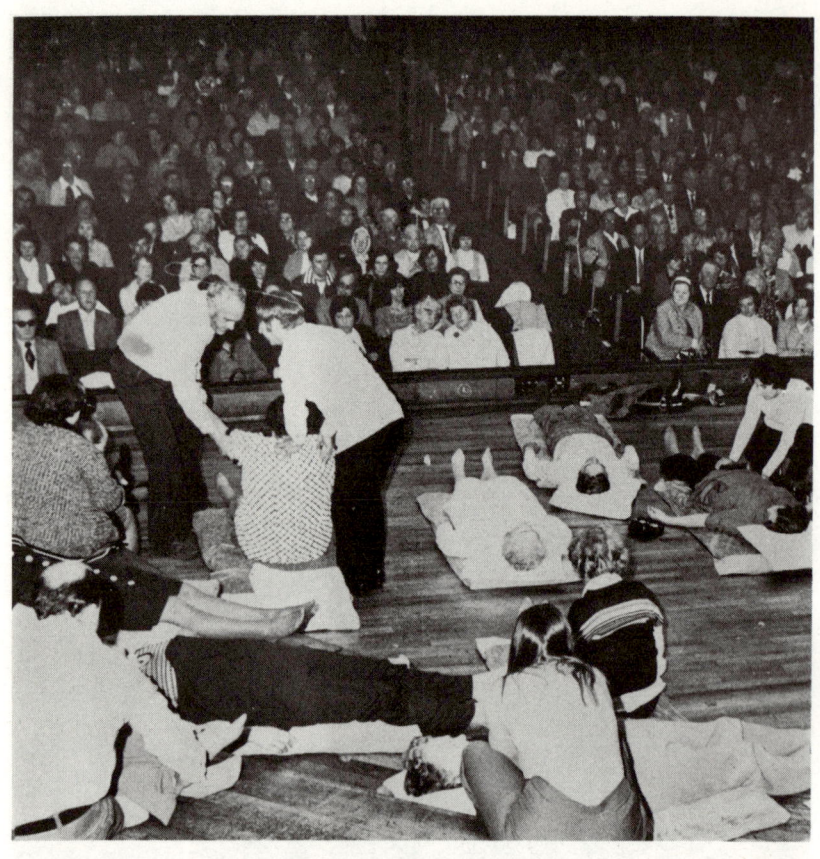

*In September 1977 John Cain gave a public demonstration of healing at the Hall of the Royal Philharmonic in Liverpool. Over one thousand people came to receive healing or see John Cain at work. Independent observers estimated that approximately one third of the audience entered into an altered state of consciousness within minutes of Cain appearing on the platform.*

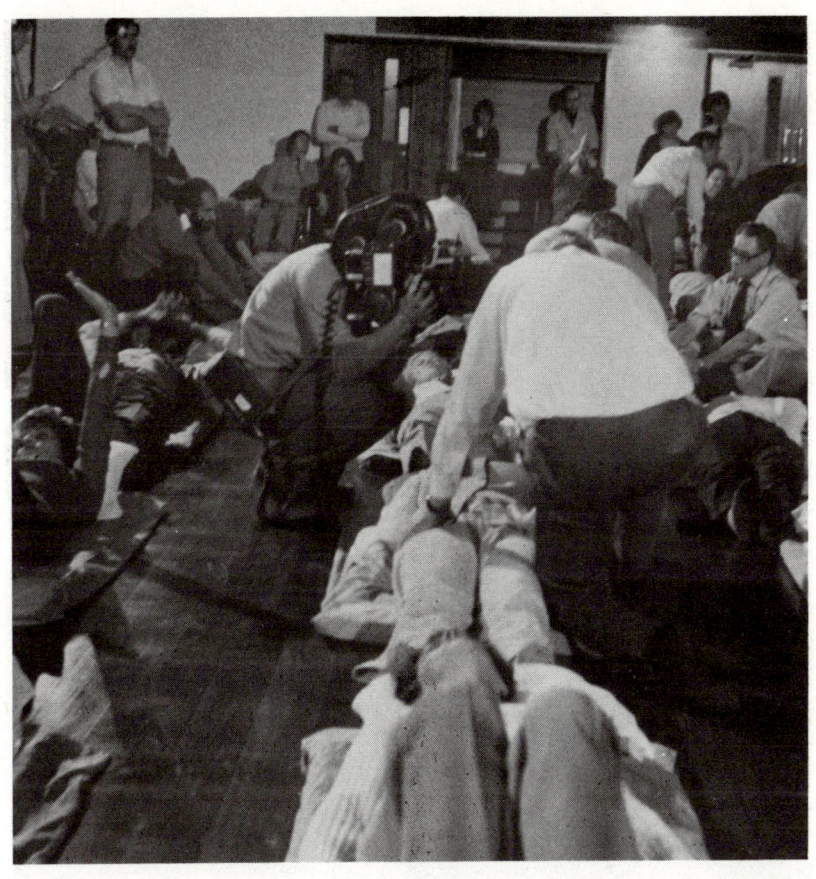

*John Cain conducts a regular clinic at Bromborough Civic Centre. In September 1979, BBC Television Glasgow sent observers there for a documentary on Healing. Producer Majorie Orr and colleagues repeated their visits several times, and they described their experiences there as 'unique'.*

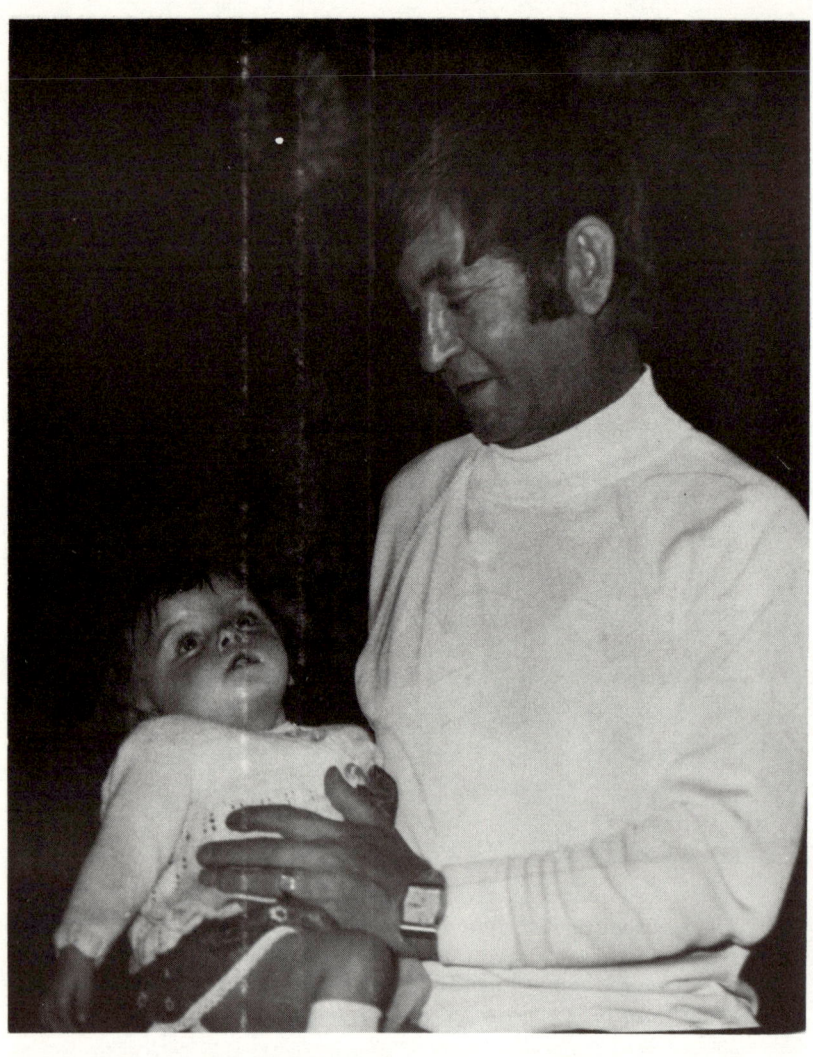

Mr. Malcolm Hughes, M.Sc., the Birmingham lecturer in psychosomatic medicine, who has made a special study of healing and who was asked by a publisher to observe John Cain during healing demonstrations, was particularly impressed by cases involving young children. "To my mind," says Malcolm Hughes, "such young children are too young to be aware of the severity of their condition or to have built up a 'faith' in John Cain to cure them."

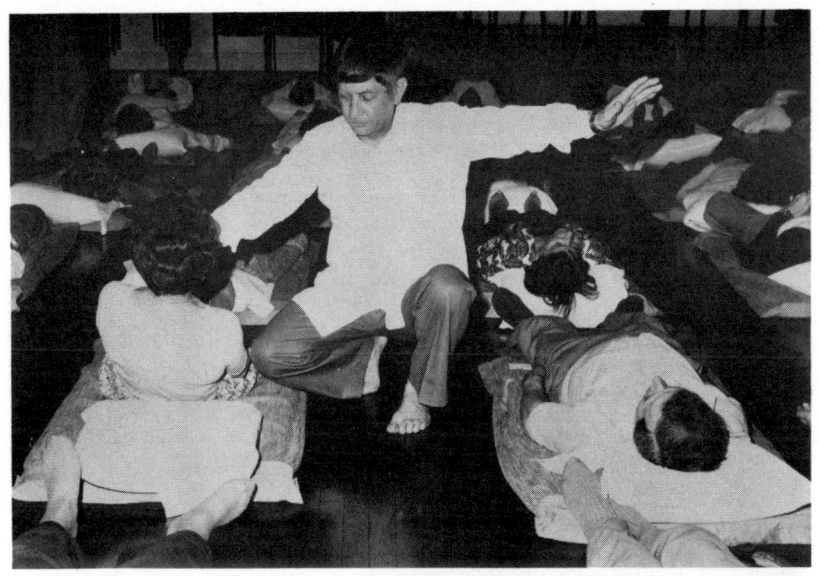

*Whilst about twenty patients are being treated in the centre of the hall, it is quite common that others, who are awaiting their turn, enter into an altered state of consciousness or even into a comatose state. Cain keeps all of them under constant observation.*

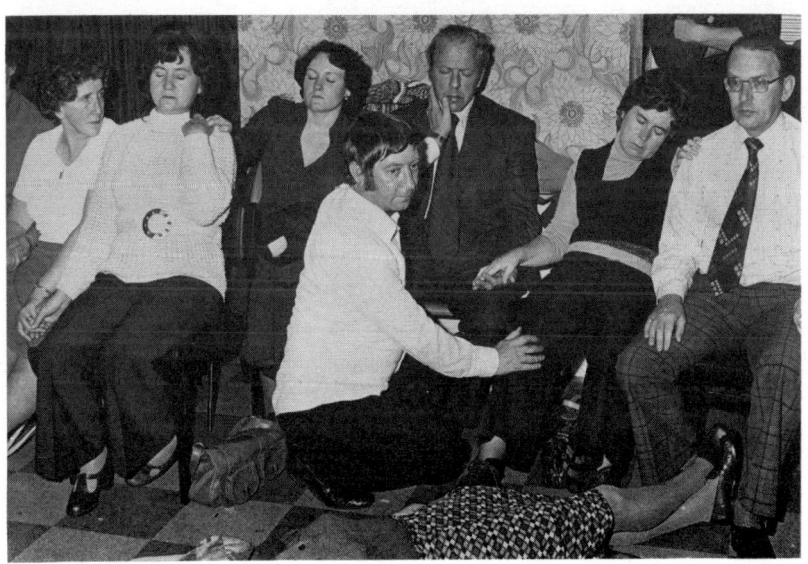

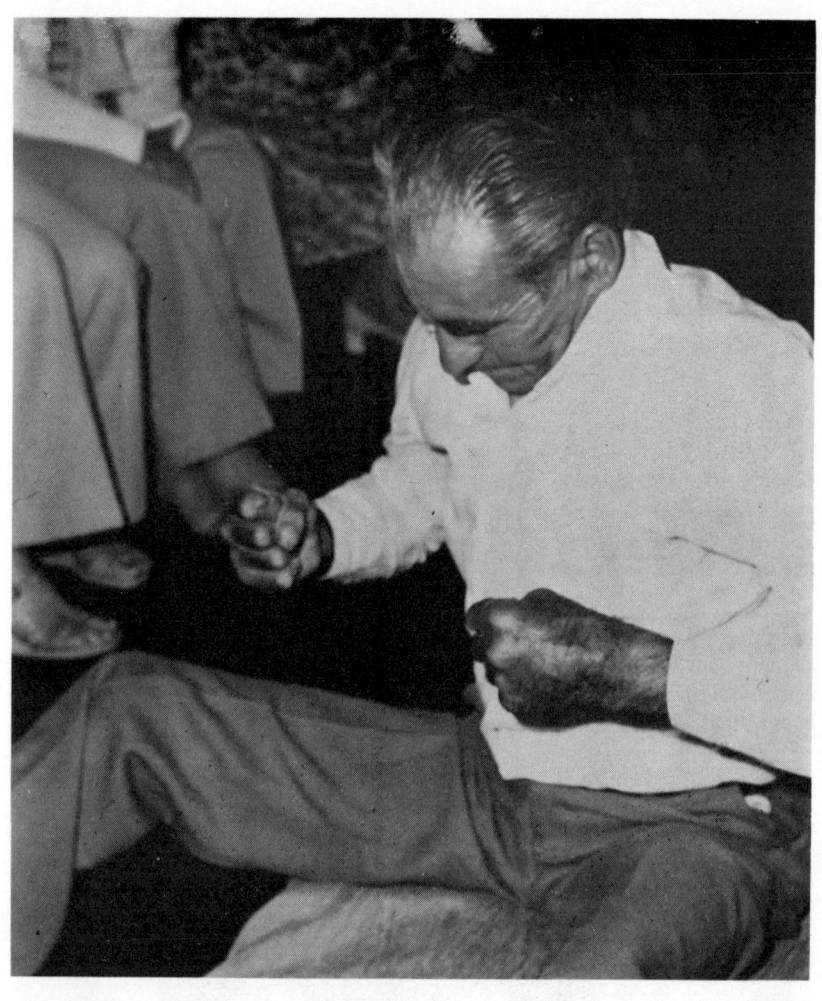

*Bill Dickinson, a sufferer from severe arthritis, tries self-manipulation in a state of altered consciousness; later John Cain offers 'resistance', requiring consider-able effort on the part of Mr. Dickinson.*

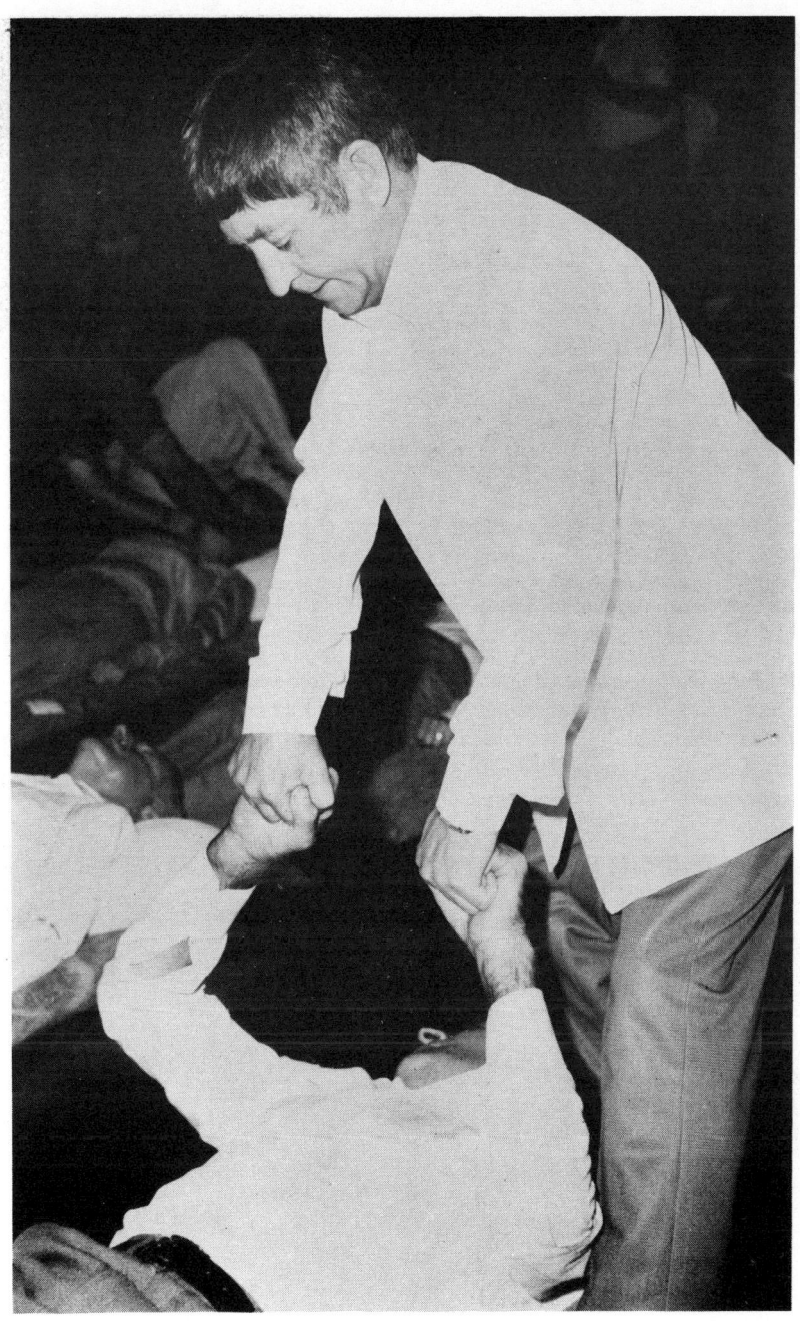

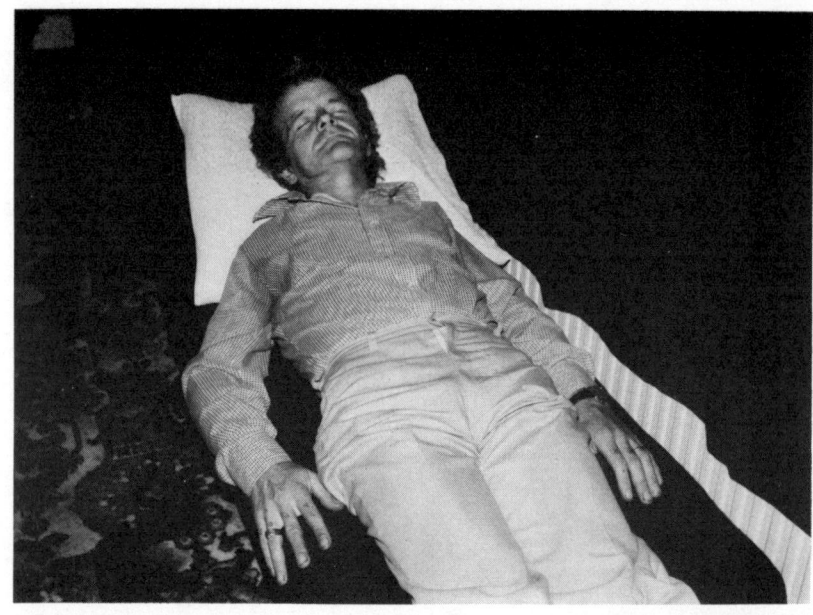

Mr. John Glover suffered an industrial accident and severely damaged his back. It was a most painful experience for him to lie down on a couch. Once he had entered into a comatose state, manipulation of the affected area took place, and these dramatic photographs of Mr. Glover's athletic feats almost belie the agony and torture he suffered when he came into Cain's room.

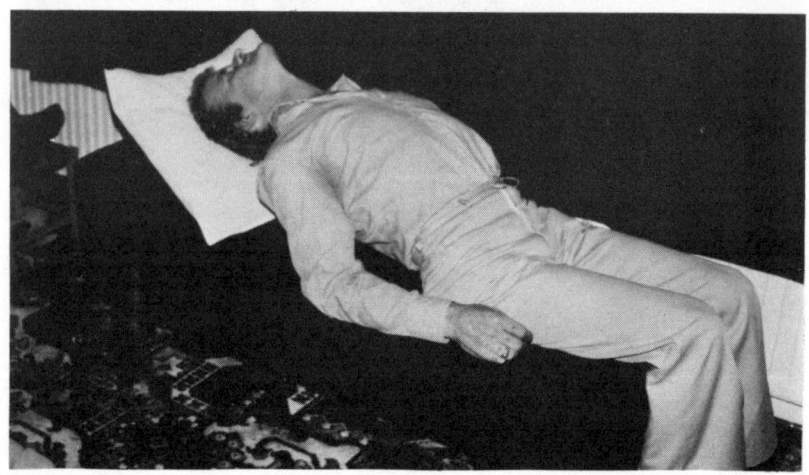

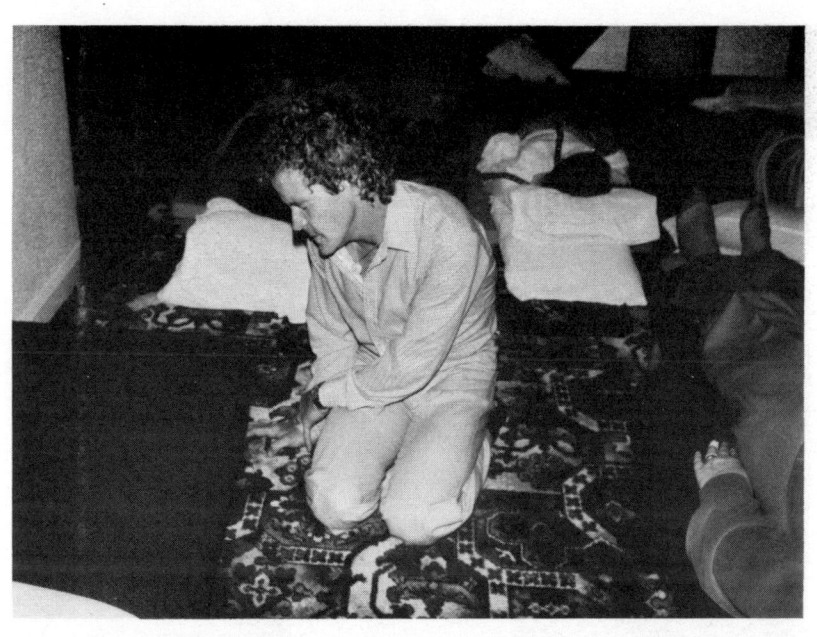

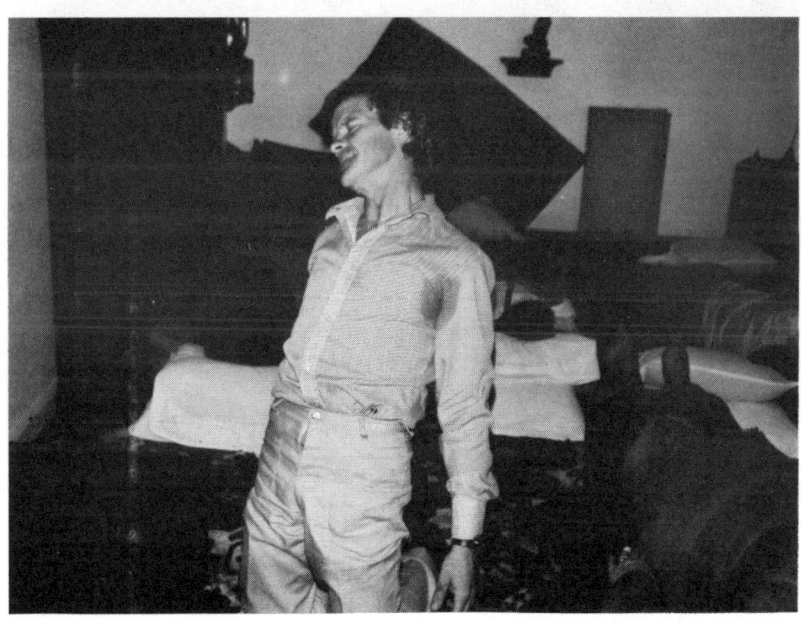

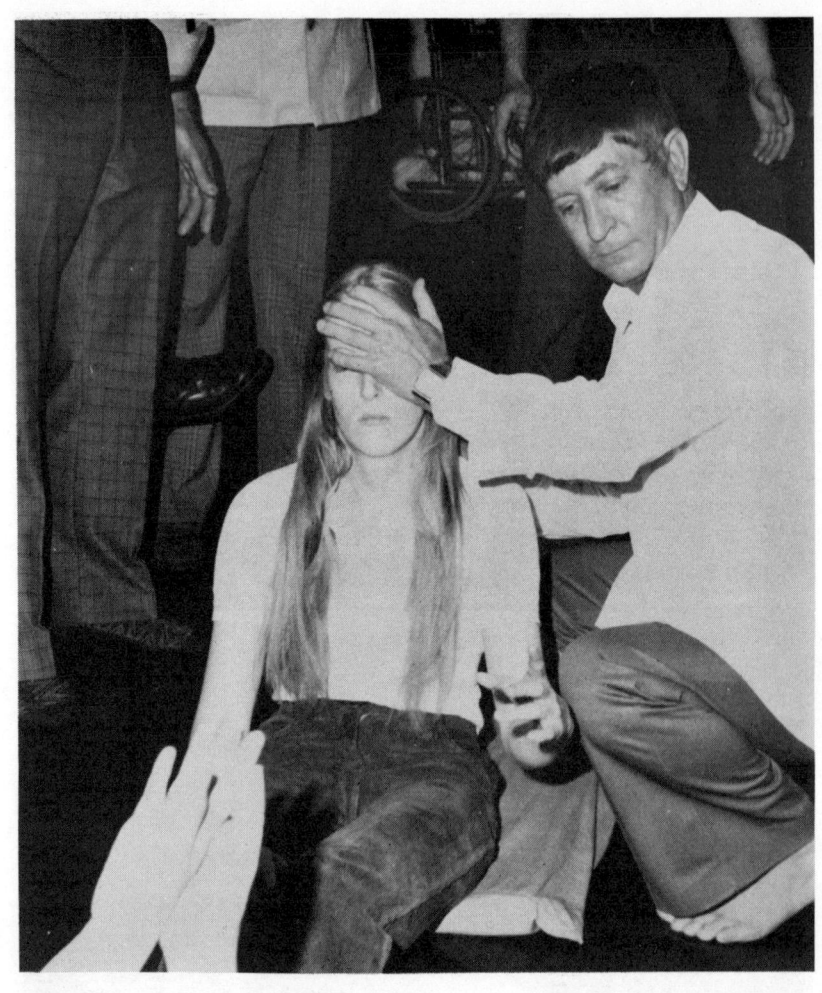

This patient has not entered into the altered state of consciousness sufficiently for the healing to take full effect. "She is one of my most difficult patients to get into a comatose state," says John Cain.

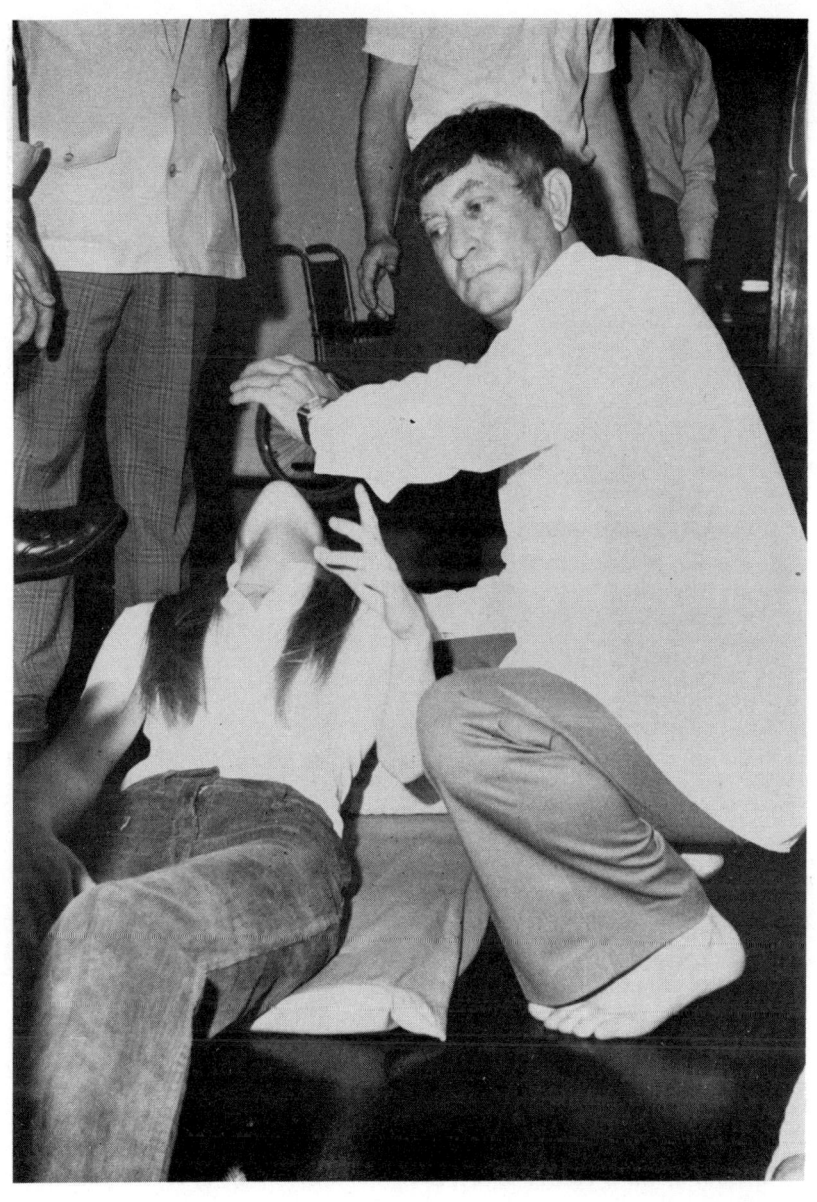

*Cain assists the patient into a deeper comatose state prior to giving her healing.*

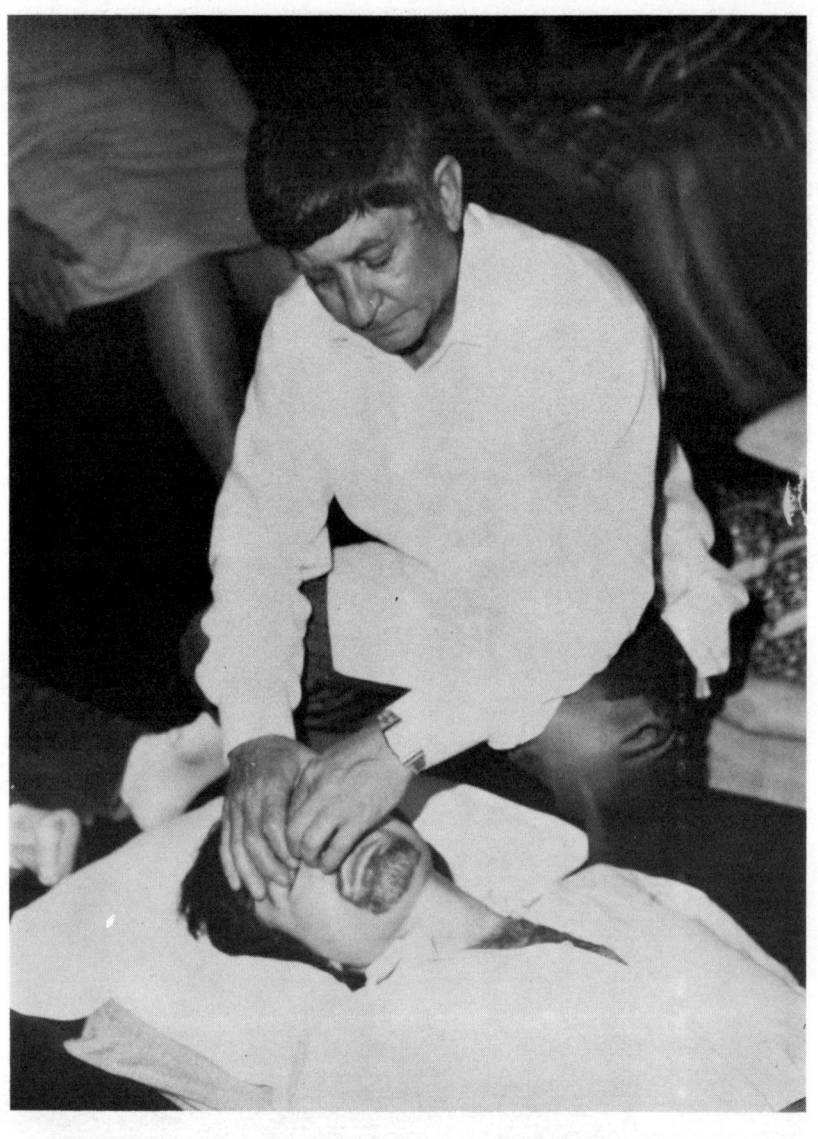

*John Cain assists a patient in deepening the altered state of consciousness.*

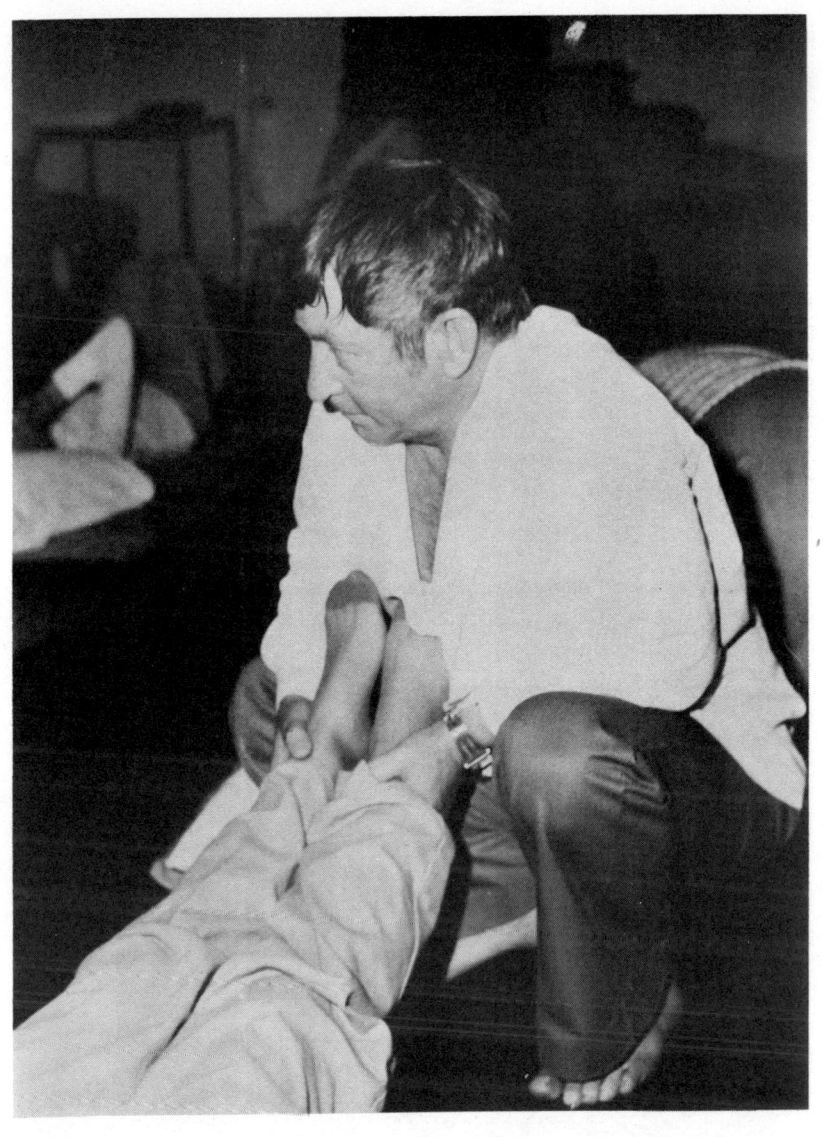

*Conditions of severe back pain are usually treated by Cain from the ankles.*

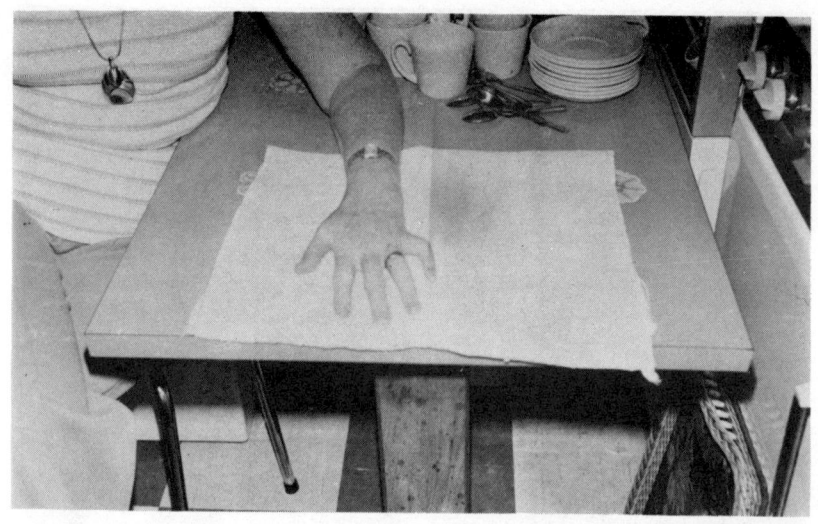

*The hand of this lady had been injured in an accident; she could not move it or close her fingers at all.*

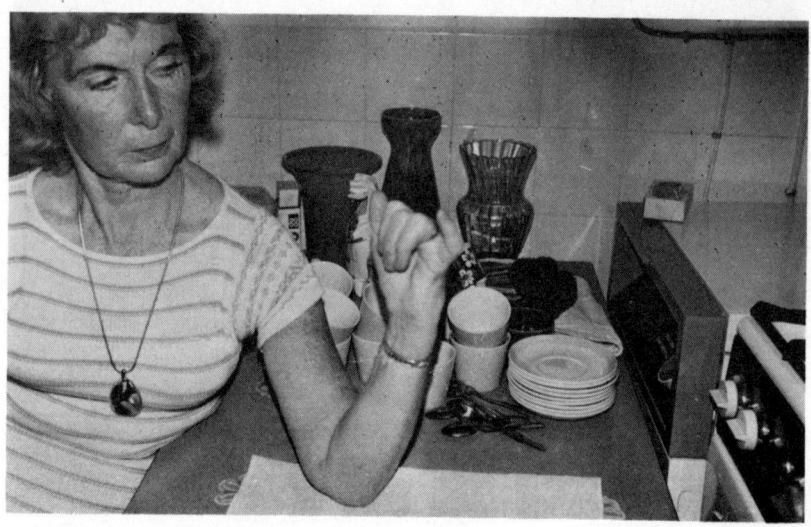

*After manipulation in an altered state of consciousness, she was able to open and close her hand and move individual fingers.*

78

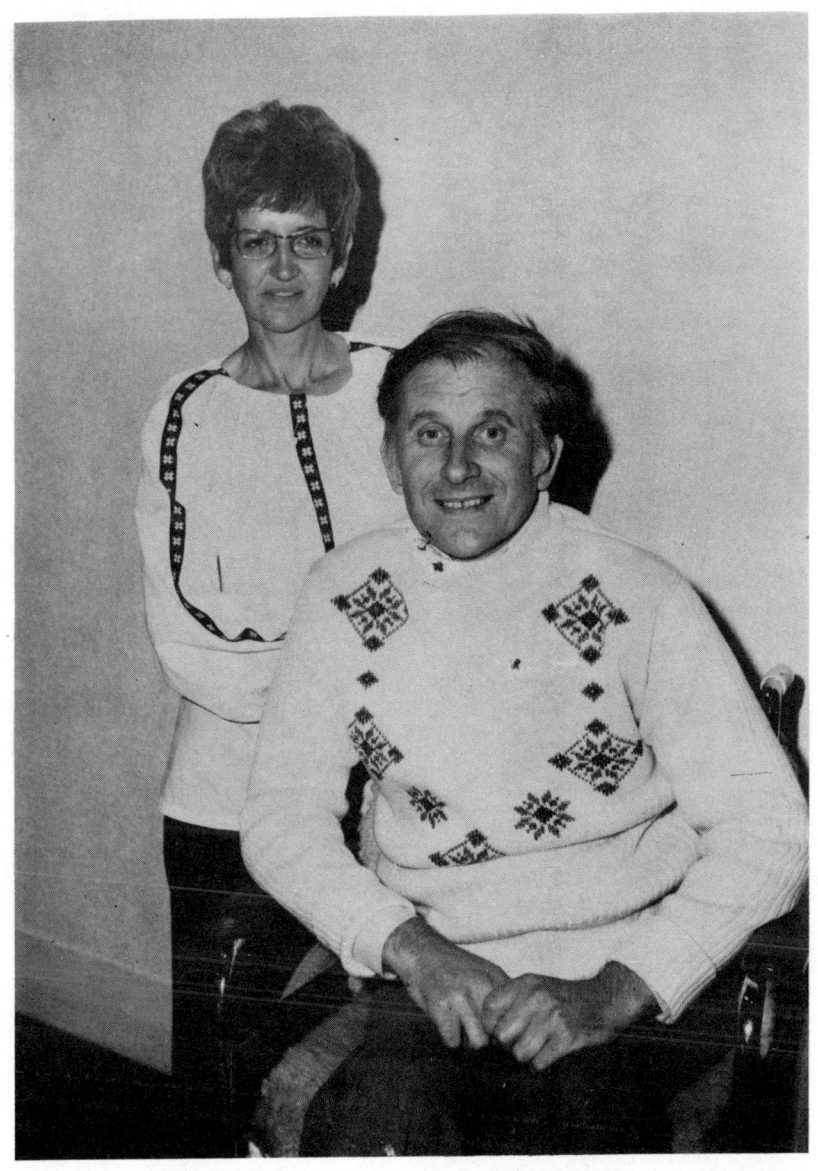

*Geoff Davies suffered severe damage to his spinal cord when a coach fell on him. After treatment from John Cain, his future looks brighter. Geoff's wife Barbara was 'conditioned' by Cain to give healing to her husband; she responded exceptionally well.*

79

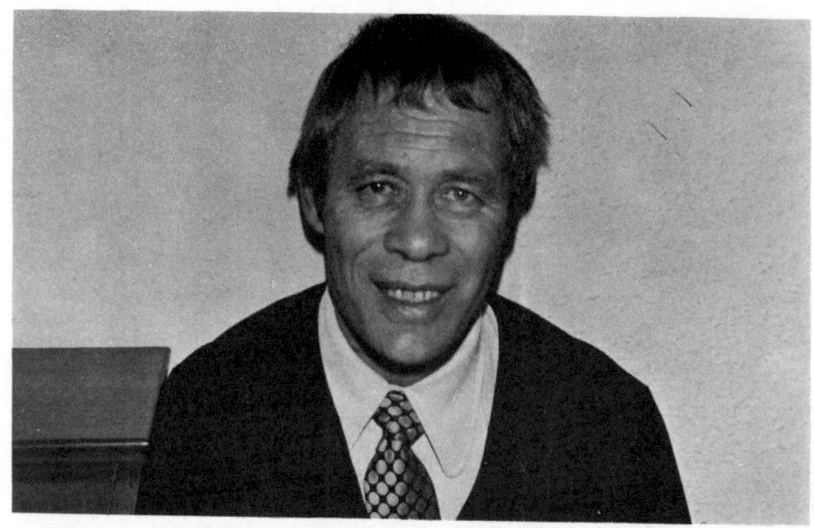

Mr. Ronald Wilson had reconciled himself to a life as an invalid, unable to write even. Over a period of one month he regained his writing ability again.

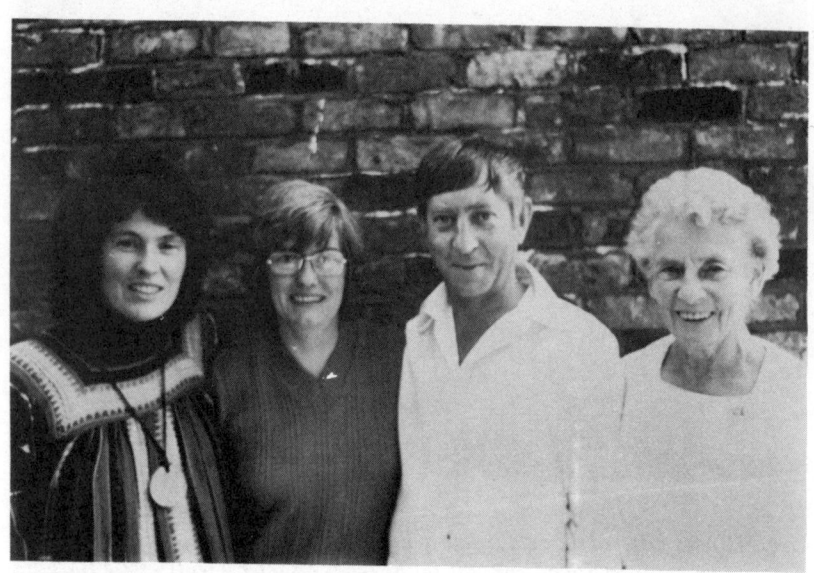

Author Pat Sykes, Audrey and John Cain, Ethel Humphreys.

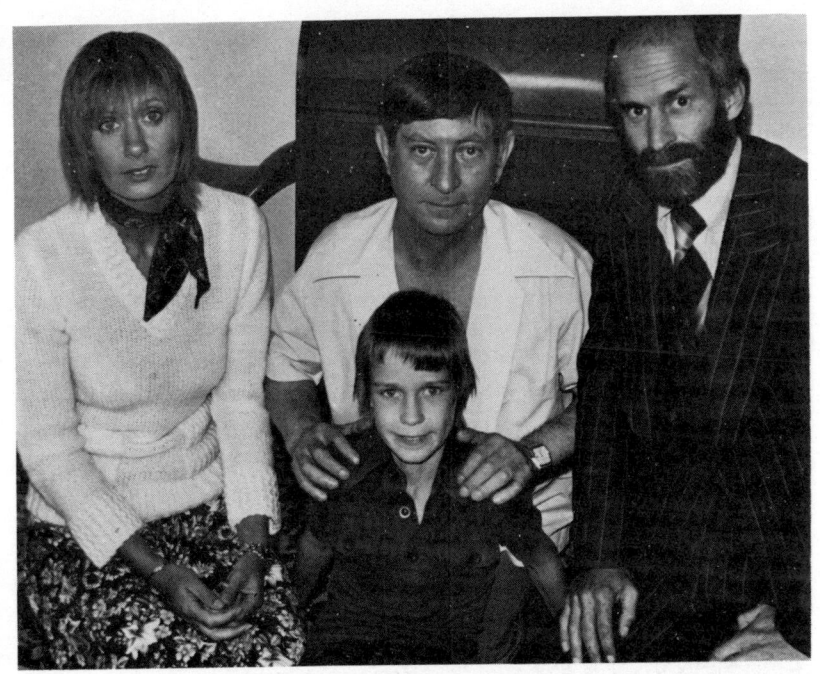

*Jason Tullett with John Cain (centre) and his parents.*

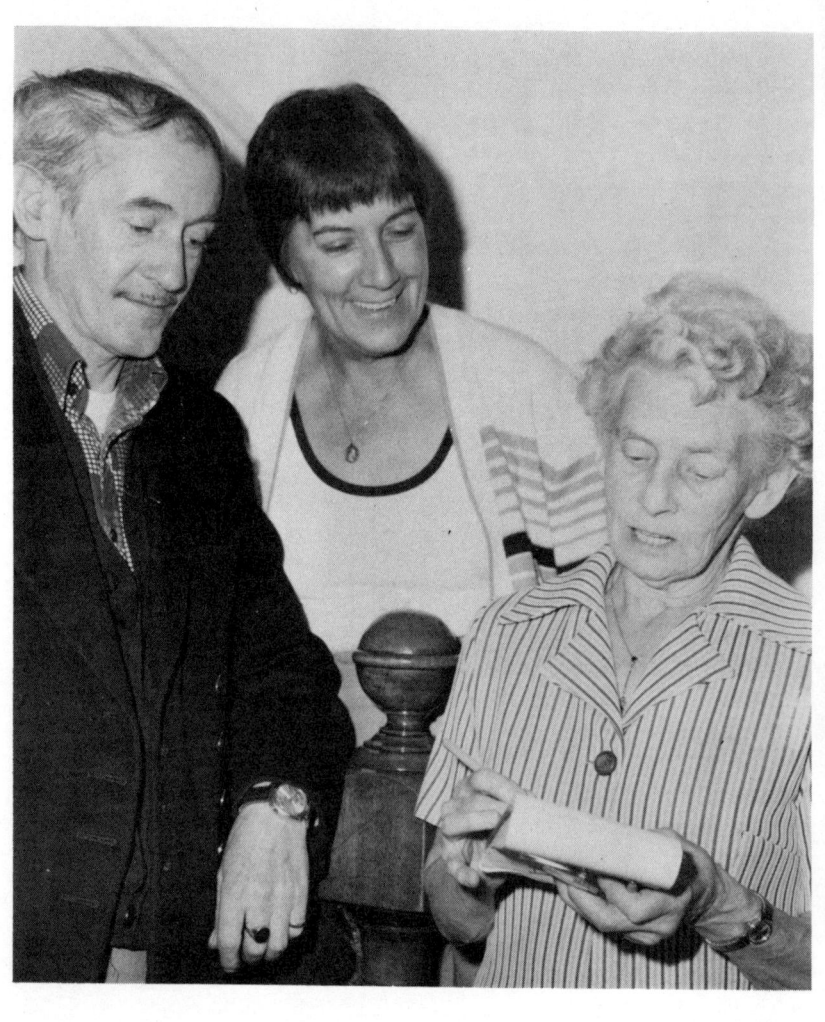

*Ethel Humphreys at reception with Douglas and Sheila Speirs, (left); John Cain during 'Absent Healing' by telephone, (right).*

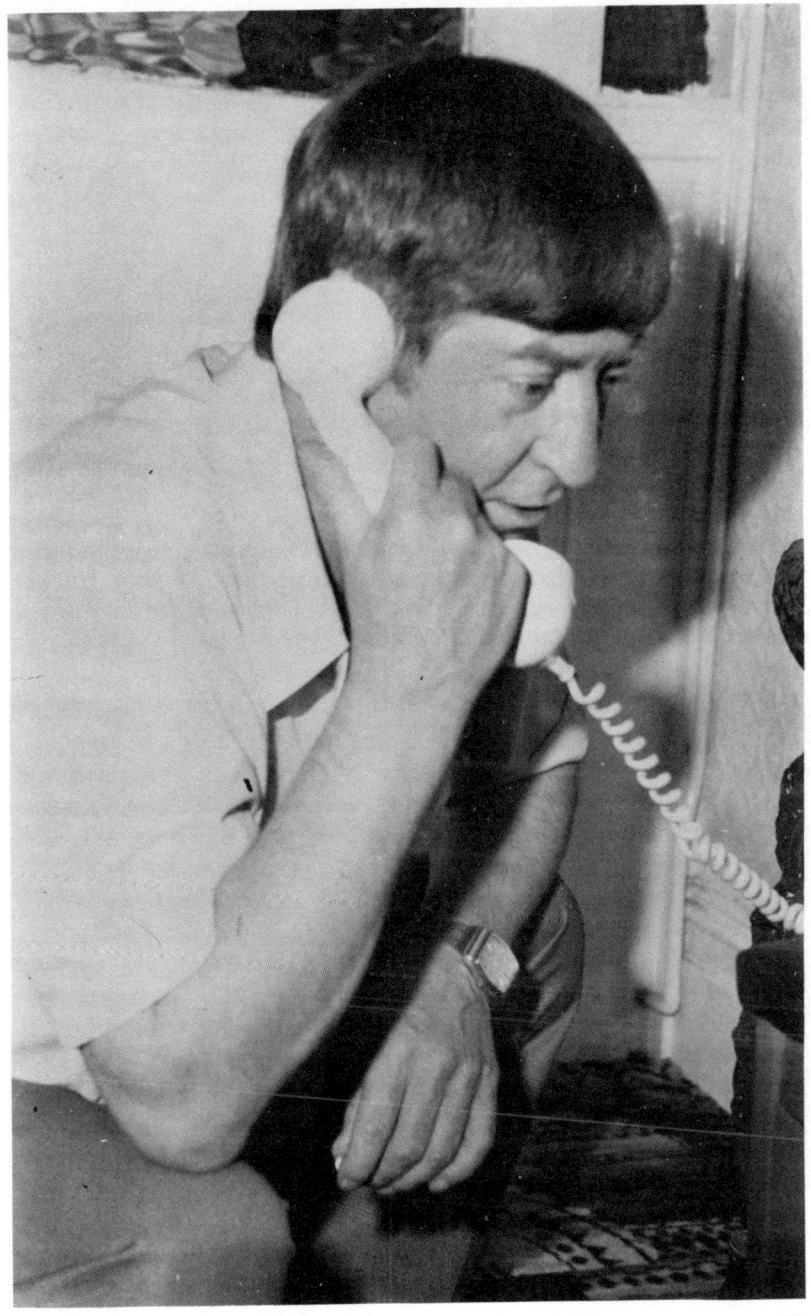

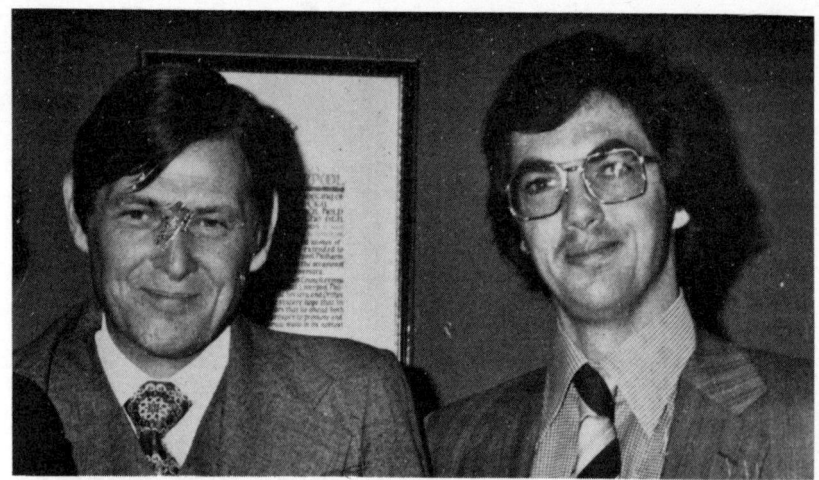

*Spiritualists and Scientists alike testify to the extraordinary gifts of John Cain. Ron Baker, former General Secretary of the SNU, and Malcolm Hughes, M.Sc., (right), were among the observers at Cain's demonstration at the Royal Philharmonic Hall in Liverpool in 1977.*

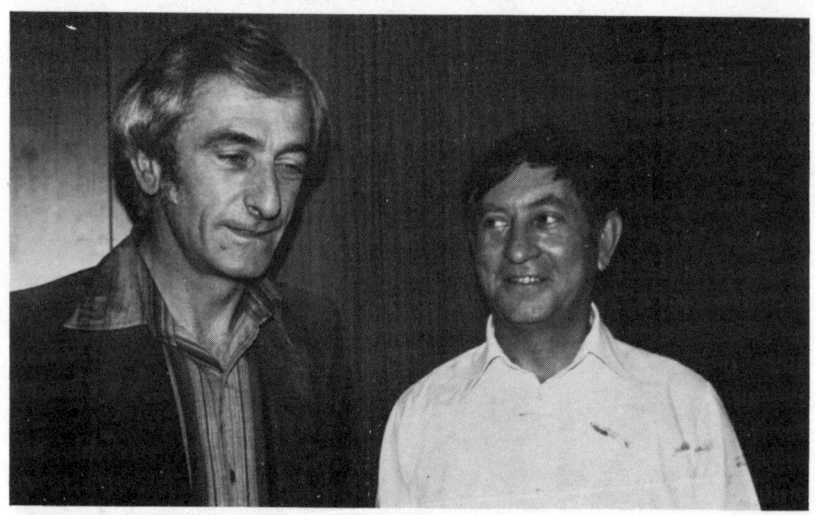

*John Cain with Mr. Jim Sword of Prenton, who came as a patient in 1977 and became a close friend of the healer.*

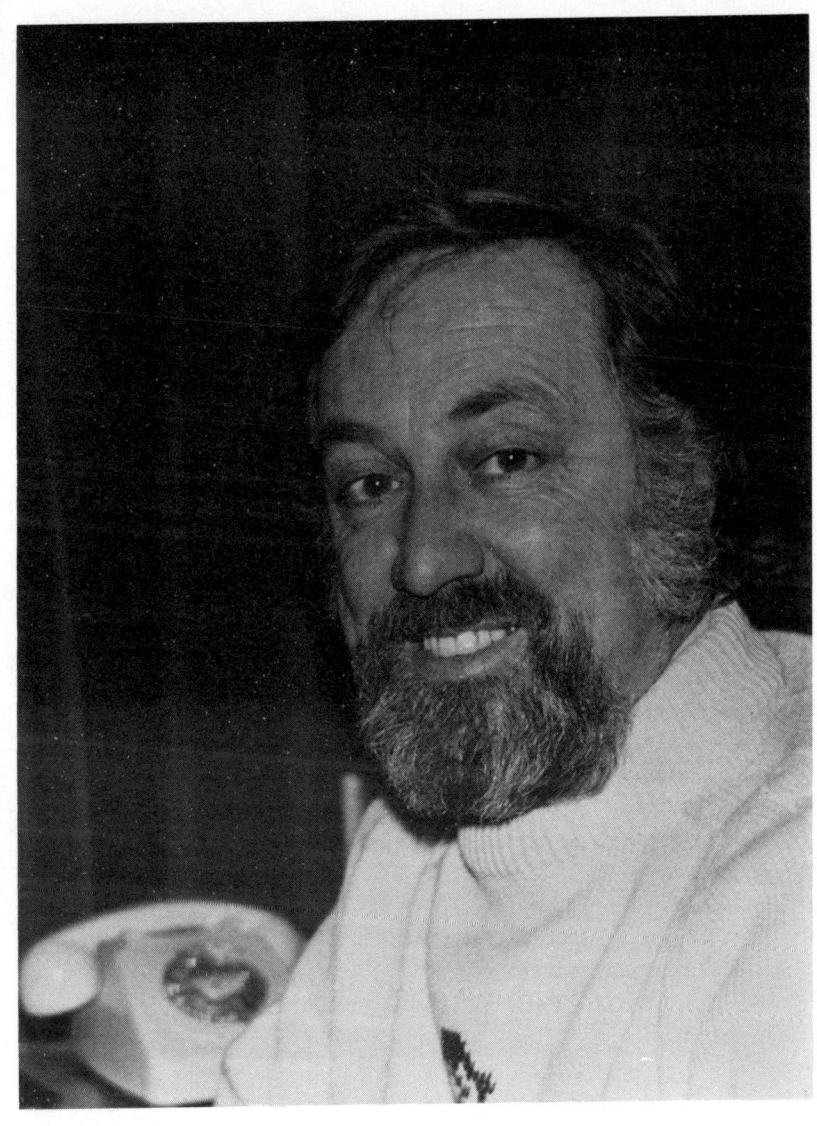

*Dr. Don Blything is one of several doctors who have studied John Cain's healing and given their verdict to the author.*

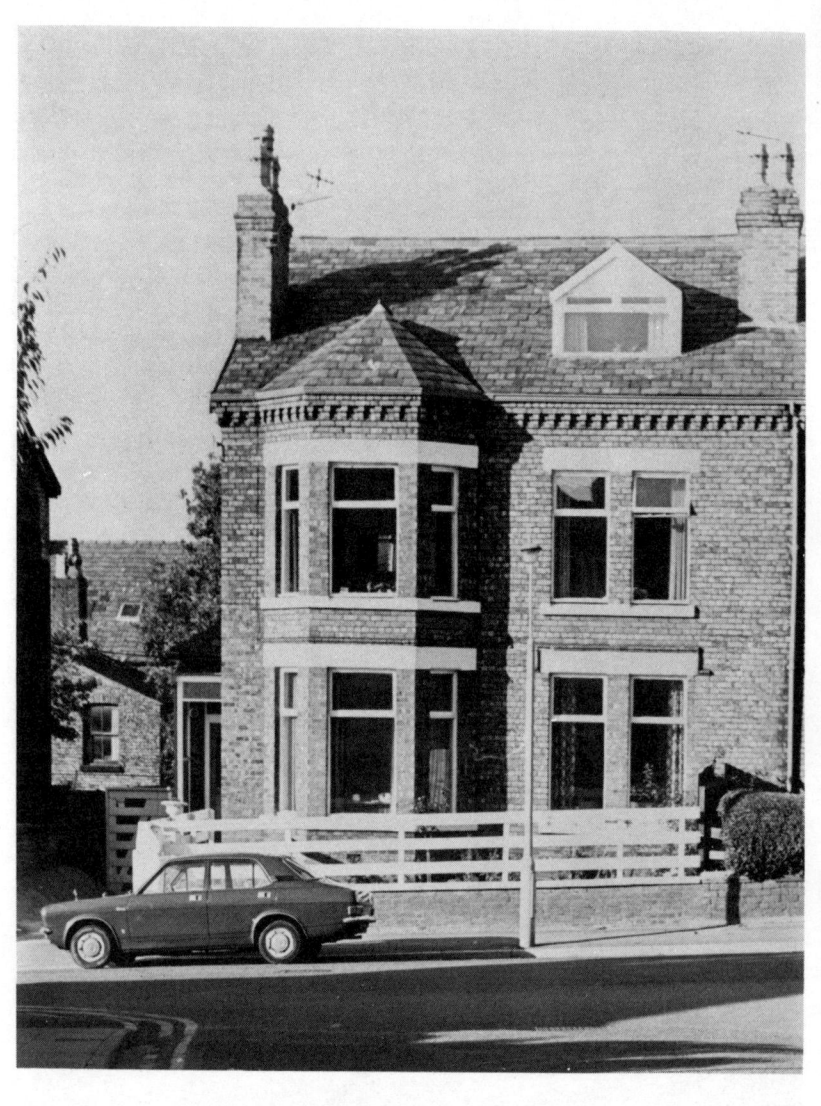

*Cain's Healing Centre in Birkenhead.*

"I was asked to 'relax' but I couldn't do so completely. John Cain came to me and laid on his hands. He lifted up my heels and the back pain which I'd had for over eighteen months left me. My arms, which I'd damaged in a works accident six years ago went 'dead' during the healing. But Cain pressed on a nerve and the feeling returned and from that time I've had no recurrence of pain either in my arms or legs."

Robert has the greatest of faith in Cain and thinks that he has given him confidence and energy to tackle jobs around the house when previously he had been unable to do the simplest of tasks. His wife, Noreen Owen does receive benefit from the healing also but her progress has been more gradual.

Robert has found that he can relax sometimes at a very deep level and although his pain has been lifted thinks the relaxation he still gets from a healing session at Cain's is very beneficial:

"I feel as if I've had a good night's sleep and am on top of the world after healing," he says.

\* \* \*

## 19.

It is difficult to measure the improvement in a condition like depression.

If someone's swollen, arthritic knees have subsided, or a skin rash or warts have disappeared then everyone agrees that there must have been some healing.

Yet there are people who have received great benefit for depression from John Cain and they are happier people because of it. The advantages to themselves and their families are enormous.

DOREEN SMITH, aged 43 from Montpelier Avenue, Weston Runcorn, first came to John Cain in April, 1979.

She had a long history of depression and sleeplessness and could not cry properly. This latter condition may seem trivial to most, but to Doreen, it was a very real problem.

After years of taking tranquilisers some of which had adverse side-effects, especially to the skin on her hands, Doreen became more and more depressed. Her future looked dismal.

Doreen had spoken to a few people who had been to Cain's and decided to go and see him. She was very apprehensive, she remembers, about what was going to happen at that first session. But, as she says: "From the moment I came through the door I felt there was a right atmosphere."

Doreen did not feel she had experienced anything at all on that first visit to Cain, except that she cried properly during the healing session. Her husband, George, though, remembers that her face showed distinct signs of being more relaxed.

After only a few more sessions, Doreen said that she felt greatly relaxed and was no longer dependant on tranquilisers.

"John Cain has lifted my depression," says a grateful Doreen. "And I think he's marvellous. For the first time in years, I now feel I'm living a normal life."

\* \* \*

I soon discovered when writing this book that John Cain does not have to bask in the glory of past healings. There are too many new healings taking place daily.

As a journalist, however, I was naturally curious to ascertain that healings had been maintained over a number of years and welcomed the opportunity to introduce a few of such long-lasting healing stories in this book.

\* \* \*

## 20.

When her friends and acquaintances see RHONA LACEY, aged 53 years, of Sutton Way, Ellesmere Port, these days, they want to know two things; why she looks so well and where have the black rings gone from under her eyes! These comments make quite a change from the ones she had grown accustomed to.

"I had suffered for twenty years with severe migraines," she told me. "My headaches were so bad that several times I'd been paralysed down my left side. 'There is no known cure', I kept hearing from doctors. And often I felt it wasn't worth being alive."

Then by chance, someone made an appointment for her to see John Cain in the days when he was healing at his bungalow. This was in November, 1974.

"I felt I had to keep the appointment even for my friend's sake, who'd been so thoughtful."

It was a decision she would never regret.

After three visits she admits she did not feel much better, except she had benefited from the relaxation experienced in the altered state. But she still kept going. "After all," she thought, "I've been going to doctors for twenty years, not feeling better, and still returning to try a different treatment, so I thought, why not give John Cain a chance?"

Then one day, whilst out shopping, Rhona felt that something had happened to her.

"The best way I can describe it," she recalls, "is that I felt as if I'd been taken out of a shell. From that day to this I have never had a serious headache again and very seldom have to take any form of tablet at all."

Rhona's healing took place over four years ago and although she cannot understand why it happened, she acknowledges that John Cain has given her a better life.

## 21.

For many years HARRY JAMES, of 48 Cleehill Road, Prenton, Birkenhead, had recurring corneal ulcers. He received treatment at an eye hospital; drops and ointment and sometimes cauterisation. The condition responded, but always it recurred.

Then, in 1972, he met John Cain at his nephew's house. Cain was treating him and whilst there was asked to see if he could help Harry.

"John Cain just placed his hands on the back of my head and then over my eyes, and although I did not feel anything in particular, my condition cleared up within days. I'm glad to report that five years have passed and my eyes are still clear."

Harry firmly believes in John Cain's healing gift and has returned to him whenever he has felt in need of healing for any other ailment; always, he says, he has received benefit.

## 22

It is always heartening to report on the successful and lasting healing of a child.

LEE ATHERTON, now aged nine, was brought to John Cain in September, 1975.

A diabetic, his daily insulin dosage was then very high; around forty units.

His father, Nigel Atherton, from Neston, Wirral, recalls what happened when Lee had healing from Cain:

"At his first healing session, Lee reported that he felt intense heat from John Cain's hands. I remember that Cain said that diabetes was a difficult condition to treat but it would be marvellous if Lee's dosage could be reduced by half.

After the session, Lee's dosage did indeed drop well below half and astonished us all. Eventually, it stabilized to around fourteen to eighteen units which he has maintained approximately for four years."

What is so striking about this story is that by rights, as Lee's food intake increases with age, his insulin dosage should increase also.

"But this has not happened," reports Nigel Atherton, "and for a diabetic he leads a remarkably healthy life. The hospital doctors are quite frankly baffled by our son's low insulin intake and our own doctor has said all along that we have his blessing to continue with the healing from John Cain."

Nigel still keeps in contact with John Cain and through Cain gives his son healing from time to time.

His son reports that always he experiences heat and a feeling of 'pins and needles' during the Absent Healing.

Nigel feels that the continued link with Cain is important for his continuing good health as he develops.

"Without Cain," he says, "I'm sure he would not be in such good condition. Other diabetic children we know about have been in hospital occasionally. Lee has never been an in-patient in four years."

When I checked details before finalizing this story in August, 1979, Lee Atherton still maintained his good health and his mother had some extra good news for me.

It seemed that since she had first spoken to me, not only had Lee's insulin dosage been reduced still further but there had been no signs of any sugar in his urine!

Mrs. Atherton had this to say about Cain:

"We place great store by Cain's healing ability and thank him for the health he has given our son."


## 23.


ARTHUR KNOWLES, from Seaforth, Liverpool, is a very tidy-minded person. He was annoyed, therefore, to see a copy of *Reveille* lying on a chair.

"That paper's been there for too long," he said in exasperation.

He picked it up, ready to tear it up, in fact, but instead, opened it at the centre spread. To this day he cannot explain why he did such a thing.

The story printed there was about John Cain.

Arthur read it and realised that this was the second instalment of a series about the healer.

Fascinated, he went in search of the first instalment and was relieved that he hadn't thrown that one away.

His daughter had a shock the same evening when she brough that week's copy of *Reveille* in and her father made a grab at it; he had always said he disliked the magazine before!

But now Arthur was interested in the publication for a very special reason.

His wife, Eileen, aged 60, had been ill for three years since it was first discovered she had three inoperable tumours. She had been told that the three tumours she had could not be removed surgically because in the first place, they had 'gone too far' and secondly, being a diabetic, it was considered too great a risk to operate on her.

Radium treatment was administered and, as far as could be ascertained, the further spread of growths had been contained. But Eileen was left with radium burns which 'wept' continually and never healed properly.

Moreover, she was still in great pain which stabbed at her back 'like a knife', she recalls, and morphine had been prescribed.

The pain, together with the poor condition of her skin, convinced her that she had not recovered from the original trouble and her spirits were very low.

She had been in this miserable condition for almost three years when Arthur first read about John Cain.

Eileen decided to go to a session at Bromborough in September, 1977, because she thought, "What have I got to lose? Time is running out for me."

She goes on to describe that first meeting:

"I can't explain it, but I knew I'd come to the right place. I didn't expect a 'cure' but I felt that somehow I'd get help here."

Eileen was very relaxed for the first few sessions although John Cain had not yet 'touched' her.

Then her husband won two tickets to attend the large demonstration at the Philharmonic Hall in September, 1977 and for the first time, John Cain himself gave her contact healing.

From that night, Eileen noticed that things began to alter:

"The angry weeping area on my breast and right hand side of my body subsided and the skin appeared more normal in colour. This caused special comment from the specialist at the Liverpool Clinic only three days after the public demonstration.

"Something's happening here!", he said, 'and in the right direction.'

"He was genuinely surprised and suggested that instead of monthly visits, I need only see him every three months."

Eileen continued to see John Cain twice a week and grew stronger and healthier and felt younger than she had for five years.

Her pain began to diminish gradually until it disappeared altogether.

The diabetic consultant was extremely puzzled that, at her check-up, a few months later, her blood now showed no trace of sugar. He commented that this can sometimes happen and suggested that she return in twelve months instead of the usual six months.

After this consultation, Eileen celebrated and bought herself a huge meringue! And from that day to this, nearly two years have elapsed. She has eaten anything she fancies. Her blood reports have always been the same: no sugar. She has even missed out a meal which is unheard of for a diabetic to do. Furthermore, any accidental cuts now heal quickly and cleanly.

Eileen was for many years a State Registered Nurse. She acknowledges that the medical treatment helped her. But she adds this: 'I was still so very ill for three years after the best medical care available and only started to become well when I went to John Cain's, that I have to say that I have had a marvellous healing from him.

"I have lived two years longer than medically expected and continue to grow in health and vigour. I have seen 'cures', during the last two years whilst attending John Cain, that all my nursing experience told me could never happen."

24.

Illness in one member of a family can cause more than a disruption in the routine; it can often break up a marriage. The stresses and strains endured by the sick person can rebound on the wife or husband. BILL and DOROTHY DICKINSON believe that not only has John Cain given them healing, but he has patched up their marriage.

Bill Dickinson, aged 52, from Ormskirk, near Liverpool, had been so crippled with arthritis since Spring, 1974 that he confesses he was very difficult to live with.

A driver by profession, he managed to keep his job but was unable to dress himself. He was not eating or sleeping and was a 'bag of nerves' with the pain. He is a slim man anyway but he lost two stone.

Hospital treatment followed after pain-killers and the drugs in common use for the relief of arthritis had failed to help him. Bill had extensive blood tests in November 1977 and returned once monthly for check-ups. His condition did not improve.

Then, the following Spring a next-door neighbour saw the *News of the World* article about John Cain and Bill traced one of the patients mentioned in it. She told him where to go and see John Cain. Bill's story from there is quite remarkable:

"My wife and I went to the Bluecoat Chambers, Liverpool, on a Saturday where there was to be a public session. Quite honestly, I was scared stiff but my wife had encouraged me to go. In any case, I was in so much pain, I thought what had I got to lose.

"I watched for a while and was in two minds about staying; the 'trances' people were going in frightened me. It was my turn to lie down and from then I don't remember a thing. Afterwards they told me what had happened. I'd just gone 'out' straight away and apparently made a terrific din. I was banging my limbs all over the place so my wife told me. I didn't even hear the music.

93

"When I awoke one-and-a-half hours later I didn't know what had happened except that night my pain had gone! I went to bed and didn't wake until 4 p.m. the next day. I ate a huge meal for the first time in years, could lift my hands above my head and my wife just cried with relief."

Bill does not need tablets or pain-killers any more and has refused any gold injections. After three months of attending John Cain, Cain said to him, "When you go to hospital they'll say you're seventy-five per cent better!"

John Cain was not far out in his predictions. The specialist asked Bill, "Do you feel as good as you look because you look eighty per cent better!"

Bill's illness and its surrounding stress took its toll on his marriage and Dorothy Dickinson left Bill in Spring, 1979.

A happier Dorothy spoke to me, though.

"The five months I was away from Bill, my health was very poor and I felt I had to come back to John Cain. In fact, Bill and I were reconciled at John Cain's house. We're not fanatics about religion or the supernormal. We needed help physically and spiritually and he was there to give it."

"Without John Cain," says Bill, "I wouldn't like to think where I'd be. I owe him my personal happiness and my livelihood."

25.

The story of DOROTHY HEWETT, aged 51 of Stanpark Avenue, Netherton, Liverpool is a good example of how Cain's clairvoyant gift can be used on occasions to assist in the healing.

Dorothy came to John Cain because she had noises in her head. She had been to four different specialists all of whom had offered different explanations for her condition but could suggest no particular treatment.

Dorothy had become very depressed although she did not reveal this to Cain but merely told him about the noises.

She explains how her whole life was changed after only one session of healing from Cain on December 22nd, 1977.

"Cain was, of course, concerned about the noises but he insisted that there was something I was hiding which was more damaging to

94

my health and happiness than the noises in my head.

"He said that only when I spoke about what was troubling me would I get well physically."

Dorothy admitted to Cain that indeed she had carried guilt around with her for over twenty years about having to return a baby, Deborah, her husband Joe and she had intended to foster.

"When Debbie was three months old, we were told she would be spastic. I was pregnant and having lost one baby, I was advised not to take Debbie on. I never got over the guilt that I should have kept Debbie."

Dorothy is a much happier person today, though. Debbie, too, now aged 23, whom Dorothy and Joe have kept in touch with, has received great benefit from Cain and visits him weekly.

"Before Debbie went to Cain's," says Dorothy, "she couldn't walk up stairs but had to slither up on her seat. Her legs were rigid. Now she climbs steps and altogether her walking is greatly improved. Cain makes no rash promises and says it will take a long time but he is confident that she will go on improving."

Dorothy is no longer depressed over Debbie, she says, and the fact that she and her husband have become helpers of Cain is one of the great blessings in their lives.

"We thank John Cain every day for the increased happiness he's brought us since we've known him," she says gratefully.


26.


To be seriously ill is bad enough; to be seriously ill and not to know what is wrong with you is a double worry.

SHEILA FYLES, aged 37, from Anglesey, North Wales, was in just this state about five years ago.

She was operated on for a stomach growth after an appalling record of ill-health: she lost her voice, could not keep food down and went down to five-and-a-half stone in weight.

After the operation, she was in hospital for twelve months and was so weak she did not walk until the end of that period, and then only with a stick. She had a shadow on her left lung, could not digest her food and was still under weight. That was when they sent her home, with the phrase ringing in her ears that has become so familiar to many sick people: 'There is nothing more we can do for you'.

Looking back, she doesn't know how she kept alive. With four children to look after, although she had help from her mother, she was in a desperate situation.

There was still a mystery surrounding her medical case and she still had the worry of that on her mind.

Then she developed lumps in her breast, neck and groin and further surgery was recommended.

That was when she made her decision:

"I'd had enough of hospitals," she said, "I'm not going to undergo any more operations for anyone."

At the same time she made this decision, she read about John Cain in the *News of the World* article and wrote off, with many thousands of other sick people, for his address.

By the time she made it to Bromborough, in June 1978, Sheila was weak, not sleeping, and not eating much except warm 'sloppy' food.

She recalls that first visit:

"I didn't expect a thing to happen and was surprised when I lay down and felt suddenly relaxed and a tingling in my legs like an electric current. I was 'out' for about an hour and when I awoke I felt hungry for the first time in years!

"I can honestly say I never looked back from that day. The lumps disappeared gradually but I was pain-free almost immediately.

"I owe my life to John Cain."

Sheila's daughter, Tracy, aged 8 years, has also received healing from John Cain.

She was rushed off to hospital in October, 1978, when she suddenly was unable to walk; had swollen ankles and was feverish. The diagnosis was rheumatic fever.

Sheila rang John Cain and he said to go back to the hospital and to tell Tracy to concentrate on him.

Tracy recovered so well that she was sent home after a few days for a trial period whilst they awaited the results of tests.

Meanwhile, Sheila continued to bring Tracy to John Cain.

The results of the tests puzzled the hospital; they had expected something to be amiss but everything showed up normal. They would not sign her off in case of a recurrence of her symptoms, and have done more tests, all of which have been all right.

At the time of writing this book, Tracy is still perfectly well.

\* \* \*

## 27

In 1976, JOAN JONES, aged 35, from Caernarvon, was given six months to live.

In July, 1979, still very much alive, she told me her story!

"It was diagnosed that I had hardening of the arteries. In fact, I was so bad they said I had the inside of a woman of eighty.

"I was given tablets to thin my blood and told to go on a strict diet and give up smoking. But I must admit, I wasn't very good at sticking to either of those suggestions and I suppose you could say I'd lost heart."

It was Joan's mother who made her come and see John Cain, and when he saw what was written on her card and how young she was to have such a condition, he just did not believe it!

Joan went into a very deep relaxed state right from the start and when she awoke one thing struck her straight away.

"I immediately thought, 'I'm no longer afraid of dying'.

"I knew I must come again and make the round trip of 170 miles once a week to see John Cain. In the week I use his photograph to relax me."

Joan reports that the hospital still cannot understand why she is still alive.

## 28

Also making the long trip weekly to see John Cain is JOAN OWEN, aged 58, from Caernarvon.

After four operations on her knee joints, Cain frankly admitted to her that he didn't think he would be able to help with her knees.

"But he has," says a thankful Joan. "I used to need a walking-aid, and now I don't need it, and although I still have pain, I can bear it because John Cain has altered my outlook on life."

Joan also telephones John Cain when she feels the need, and once, she related that when she had an attack of breathlessness, which is something that bothers her from time to time, she started to dial on her wall 'phone. However, she only got as far as the code for

Merseyside and had to sit down, still holding the 'phone because of her condition. When she felt stronger, she tried to complete the dialling. Before she had chance to dial any more numbers, to her utter amazement, she recognised John Cain's voice! He was talking to a reporter.

"I thought I was going mad," recalls Joan, "but I plucked up courage and said, 'John, can you hear me?' He said, 'what on earth are you doing on this line?' and was as surprised as I was. I heard the reporter say, 'Shall I go off,' but Cain said, 'no, stay and listen to this.' He then told me to lie on the bed and he would 'phone me back."

Needless to say, Joan was much better when Cain kept his promise and made that call!

29.

There is one veterinary surgeon in Minera, near Wrexham in Denbighshire, who is amazed at the recovery of one of his patients!

'Shep', a two-year-old sheep-dog became totally blind in 1973. His owner, Marie Adams, of Minera, was very distressed.

"He was such a young dog and I didn't want him to be put down. The Vet just didn't think there was much hope at all.

"Anyway, I had heard of Mr. Cain and have always had an open mind about healing so thought I would take Shep to him."

Marie took Shep and John Cain conducted a healing session on his eyes and said to Marie, "He will see in about ten days' time."

Cain was not far out in his prediction!

After two weeks Shep suddenly got his sight back and Marie rang her vet. She didn't tell him the good news immediately but asked him, "do you think that Shep will ever get his sight back?"

"To be honest," he replied, "It would be a miracle if he did."

Then Marie broke the news to him and he was very interested and asked her to bring Shep in for confirmation. She left it a couple of weeks because the dog had become nervous whilst blind. When he saw the dog, the vet thought it was marvellous.

That was six years ago, and when I checked with Marie she told me that Shep was still in good health and had even had another healing from John Cain; this time an absent one.

"He was involved in an accident and badly injured his hip joint. I rang Mr. Cain and he said he would ask for the muscle to be strengthened. Shep very soon began jumping all over the place and was his old self again."

There is another little story to add here.

When Marie first took Shep six years ago, she was accompanied by her friend, Mrs. Thelwall, from R␡abon.

She told Cain that she had suffered for years from acute stomach pains after major stomach surgery. He laid his hands on her painful area and almost immediately her pain disapperared. There has been no recurrence of her severe pain in all those years.

Marie Adams herself has had healing on two occasions from Cain.

"Once," she told me, "he gave me treatment for nervous trouble and on that occasion I went into a deep sleep. I have never looked back from that day. Also, he replaced a disc in my neck and the pain left me immediately!"

\* \* \* \* \*

When I spoke to Mrs. Adams to check the details of her story, I was able to give her Cain's new address. This happened many times whilst writing this book; so many people had lost contact with him and were delighted to know he was still in the area.

## 30.

RONALD WILSON from Eccleston Park, Prescott, Liverpool, has always believed that one day he would be cured.

At 46, he could not believe that he had no future other than that of an invalid, but that was how it appeared to him until he came to John Cain.

An inflamed nerve at the base of his neck had affected his left leg and caused tremors in his right arm, making writing impossible.

For about four years the muscles in his calf had not been working and he dragged his toe along instead of lowering his heel, a condition

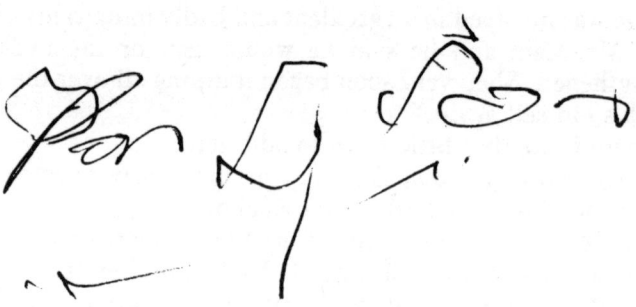

*On 22nd July 1979, Mr Wilson was unable to write his name.*

recognised medically as 'foot drop'. He was not in pain, thankfully, but his life was very restricted as he could not walk far.

Medical treatment had consisted of cortisone injections whilst in hospital for ten weeks with the injections continuing at a reduced level when he was discharged.

But the doctor's prognosis was not very good: at the most he could expect only temporary relief from the injections. He had to face the possibility that some day he would have to give up his job as a personnel manager altogether.

He heard about John Cain from a relative in 1978 but Ronald was very sceptical and thought that Cain was probably a very good masseur but could not help his condition.

Ronald saw his relative again at the end of June 1979 and decided he would give Cain a try. By then, he was in a bad way and thought as so many people who've tried everything in an attempt to get better and failed, 'what have I got to lose?'

That first visit to Cain's healing session at Bromborough is engraved on Ronald Wilson's mind for ever:

"It took John Cain's son and my parents about twenty minutes to get me into the building, even though I wore a leg support," recalls Ronald. "Cain told me he'd put me into a relaxed state. I did feel relaxed very quickly and could only hear things in the distance; my eyelids were heavy. I was aware of being prodded in the nerves of my foot and leg. I remained in this state for about an hour. Afterwards, when I came to leave I found that I could put my heels down properly and didn't need my leg support. I have never worn it since."

Ronald's condition improved steadily after this first visit and on the many occasions I saw him at Cain's centre throughout the Summer of 1979, I witnessed this improvement. He manipulated his

100

> I testify to the truth and
> accuracy of my treatment with
> John Cain and give my full and
> unreserved permission for its use
> and publication.
>
> *[signature]*
>
> 27. 8. 79.

*Since then, there has been further improvement in Mr. Wilson's ability to write.*

arms and legs more vigorously at each session whilst in the 'altered state'.

After three weeks Ronald reported that his walking had improved beyond recognition. Certainly I watched him walk into John Cain's centre without any support and more steadily with each visit. I was there on July 23rd, 1979, the day he wrote his signature whilst in the altered state and thereafter saw the attempts on paper he made at home, often again whilst in an altered state, to regain his writing ability.

Ronald Wilson's specialist commented in August, 1979 that he was walking a lot better and the use of his right arm had improved quite beyond his expectations.

At the time of this book going to print, Ronald was able to say that after only four months' healing from John Cain he could now drive his car, his arm was less tremulous and his writing almost back to normal; he could eat unaided and walk well over a mile!

"I am very optimistic about the future," Ronald says. "I am now looking forward to returning to work. Thanks to John Cain I feel that I just need to gain more confidence in my walking and that I know he will give me.

"I came as a sceptic, but now I have every confidence in John Cain as a healer because my personal experience has proved that he is totally genuine."

## 31.

Those of us lucky enough to get through life without prolonged pain can probably never fully appreciate how debilitating pain can be. JOHN GLOVER, aged 39, from Airdale Close, Ford Estate, Birkenhead, was in constant back pain as a result of an accident at work. He had little sleep for four years.

He had traction, and his pain went, only to return at the end of the treatment; he was encased in plaster for three months but had no pain relief at all.

"I was thoroughly miserable," says John. "I had no job; my family were suffering because of me. It was difficult to keep the marriage stable."

John's discs were pronounced all right but there was still a mystery surrounding the pain in his back.

In May, 1979, during the course of one week, John Glover, now nearly at the end of his tether, saw John Cain's name twice. His wife, Pat, saw it as a sign and suggested that at least he should 'give Cain a try'.

So, in June, 1979, a very nervous John Glover came to Cain's centre.

"When I saw other people lying down and going into what looked like a deep sleep, I thought, 'no way is that going to happen to me!' But it did! Not only did I relax, but after John Cain had touched my spine and held my heels, all the pain left me." John Glover was very puzzled at what had happened to him and didn't really believe anything had taken place.

He decided he must pay Cain a second visit.

"I relaxed very deeply again," he reports, "and my pain, which had returned slightly, left me again. I really believed that something wonderful had taken place".

At each subsequent healing session, John Glover self-manipulated more vigorously and did exercises which his specialist insisted he could only do under anaesthetic!

Cain asserts that because John Glover is very 'receptive', there is a strong 'fusion of minds' between the two of them during the healing.

"This enables Glover," says Cain, "to do very beneficial exercises not under his conscious control."

Cain is never afraid that Glover will hurt himself and indeed Glover reported to me after several strenuous healing sessions, that although he was often stretched very vigorously in a healing session, he has always felt 'marvellous' afterwards. I have witnessed Glover bending almost double forwards and even backwards. Once, I saw him place his palms almost flat on the ground in front of him. The specialist has been trying to get him to touch his toes for four years without success!

John Glover told me that although he is not completely free from pain in his back, he can now live with the level of pain he has, and sometimes there are days when he has no pain at all. He says: "I can now do things which had become impossible. I can decorate, drive the car without pain and I no longer take pain-killers. If I do have a flare-up, I can get almost instant relief from looking at John Cain's photograph and going into the altered state.

"I can't speak highly enough of Cain. This man wants me to get well and can't give enough time to me. Hospitals should be asking him to go in and work alongside their medical staff to help ease pain and to give spiritual comfort to the very ill."

I witnessed also the straightening of one of John Glover's fingers, damaged fourteen years ago and so stiff that he could not make a full fist properly.

He remained in a fully conscious state whilst Cain conducted the healing on his finger. Cain requested 'the intelligence' which works through him to straighten the finger completely. It was quite obvious watching the healing, that Glover could do nothing to prevent his finger from straightening and he was able in a few minutes to bend and straighten his finger without any trouble and make a complete fist! This took place in July, 1979, and numerous enquiries I made following this healing always produced the same answer, 'yes the finger is perfectly all right'. Pat Glover, John's wife, aged 36, also received a wonderful healing from Cain.

As a result of childhood injuries, she had her knee caps removed in adulthood. Her movement was very restricted and she dragged her legs going up stairs and could only come down stairs sideways. When she went to Cain's she had only thought of observing and did not really expect any healing for herself.

Her husband mentioned his wife's condition to Cain and he came to speak to her. Pat recalls what happened:

"John Cain placed one of his photographs on my knee. Immediately, I felt the bones contracting tightly. Cain then told me to straighten my left leg out but I said it was impossible and I hadn't done that for three years. Cain said, 'who said you can't?', and the next thing I knew I was standing up without support from anything which was unheard of for me.

"My legs felt like a new pair when I left his centre!"

Pat Glover reported how she maintained steady progress after that first healing session and after only a few weeks could cross her legs one over the other with no trouble at all. She also testified how much happier life became for herself and her husband as a result of the contact with Cain:

"I feel different," she says, "and have more patience with the children and seem to be able to communicate with my family better than ever before. John and I both feel we've more time for everyone socially now. We can't thank John Cain enough and think that his work is most important."

## 32.

"You had better learn to adapt yourself."

These were the hospital's final words to GEOFF DAVIES, aged 44, of Philwen, Pontybodkin Hill, Mold, North Wales.

Adapting meant learning to live in a wheelchair for the rest of his life, paralysed from the navel downwards and in constant pain. Geoff, a coach operator, was fixing the underside of a coach in 1976 when it fell on him. If he had lain still it might have been possible to winch the coach off him. As it was, his basic human instinct to free himself made him try and wriggle free causing the body of the coach to pin him down further. The result was, according to two hospitals, a severed spinal cord.

Since his first visit to John Cain's in March, 1979, there has not only been relief of his pain, but also such an improvement in his mobility that it is now questionable in John Cain's mind, and backed also by a visiting German doctor, if indeed the spinal cord was completely severed.

But I go too fast, because Geoff's story is so remarkable that every detail should be recorded. I have been fortunate enough to see Geoff twice weekly and so I have seen for myself the improvement in his condition, and at the time of this book going to print, the healing is a continuing process.

Before Geoff came this was the picture: he was seeing a specialist every six months and then every twelve months; there was no physiotherapy or occupational therapy (this had stopped when he left hospital); there were no doctor's visits, unless Barbara, Geoff's wife, requested a call and although there were district nurses even they admitted that they were learning from Barbara how to deal with Geoff. They were very much on their own.

He was on eight pain-killers a day and nights were a nightmare; the alarm having to be set every three hours so that Geoff could be turned to prevent pressure sores. With three young children to look after as well, Barbara had her work really cut out.

Geoff still tried to keep an interest in his coach business and could do telephone work, but depression at times was natural as also was the strain on their marriage.

Then a cousin of Geoff's suggested he should see John Cain. The hospital had suggested an operation to sever nerves which might or might not relieve his pain. "Try John Cain before the operation," his cousin begged Geoff. But Geoff was sceptical and it was weeks before he made up his mind to come.

That Thursday in March is one day he will never forget.

"As soon as I came into John Cain's house, I felt relaxed," Geoff recalls. "I felt very nervous and didn't know what to expect. I really thought that all the people there had been asked to come to convince me that John Cain was genuine; I thought it a 'set-up' in other words. I watched them going 'out' into the altered state, and thought all the time, 'it just isn't possible'. But then something happened to change my mind. There was a child there, aged about two, and I saw her going into a relaxed state. That gave me confidence because I knew she couldn't be putting on an act for me!

"I allowed myself to be relaxed and experienced a burning sensation in my ankle and then in my knee. I was amazed at feeling anything in my legs at all.

"A strange thing happened in the room; my pain was transferred to a girl who was very receptive; that puzzled me. My pain had not disappeared when I got home but I felt very relaxed and the car journey home was the most comfortable one I'd had since the accident."

From this point and over the following months there was continuous progress in his mobility, but most striking of all was the relief from his pain and the fact that Geoff and his wife now both slept through the night with Geoff able to turn himself.

The consultant at the orthopaedic hospital in Oswestry, Salop, expressed great interest in June 1979, about Geoff's healing treatment at John Cain's. It made headlines in the local papers and only time will tell just how interested the hospital may turn out to be. Unfortunately there is still a barrier between the medical profession and unorthodox methods which often produce inexplicable results. It appears that we must always have answers which are proved scientifically, yet paradoxically, we sometimes appear to be taking retrograde steps despite all our claims to progress.

Barbara Davies proved very receptive and was able to help Geoff at home. She was 'conditioned' by John Cain at his healing centre. At home, she played taped music to help create a peaceful atmosphere and at the link-up time for Absent Healing, 7 pm each evening, or at any time she felt necessary, she was able to assist in Geoff's healing.

At home, she reported that Geoff self-manipulated his limbs and exercised strenuously as he did at Cain's centre. In fact, it was a marvellous sight to see this man, who had been condemned to a life of near-immobility, stretch and arch his back, lift his legs, stand up in his wheelchair and even get out of it and crawl! He did all this whilst in an altered state when there was no way possible he could have done anything like it whilst fully conscious. Hypnotism? John Cain didn't even have to go near him for Geoff to go into an altered state. All I can say, is that at each healing session when I observed Geoff Davies, he grew stronger and attempted more and more strenuous exercises. And most remarkable, he reported to me that the feeling was coming back and moving down his torso.

He achieved more than a relief from his pain. After four years of suffering, Barbara Davies said they didn't expect any more than some relief but what happened was a bonus.

"Our future is brighter," she says, "and whether Geoff walks again is beside the point, although we never give up hope."

106

One day maybe I shall have the privilege of reporting that Geoff Davies has indeed walked.

33.

JOHN TULLETT, of North Road, Birkenhead, says of John Cain:
"When he took away my son's pains with one telephone call, I felt how much more could this man do with personal contact!"

The story of that telephone call made in November, 1977 makes astonishing reading and could well one day make medical history.

JASON TULLETT, then aged 9 years, had been operated on after a brain scan had revealed a large malignant growth with a cyst. It was decided that it was too dangerous to remove the growth and only an investigatory operation had been carried out.

Jason was in Walton Hospital and by his bedside when he came out of the anaesthetic were his parents, John and Sandy, his grandmother and Lizette, his aunt; always very close to her nephew, she had insisted on being there at the hospital.

At precisely 7 p.m., the four adults watched helplessly as Jason fought to conquer overwhelming pain, feverishness and an ever-rising temperature.

His breathing was rapid and frequent pain-killing injections did nothing to calm him.

His parents were distracted.

John Tullett, quite out-of-the-blue, asked his wife's mother to telephone John Cain. They had heard of him prior to Jason's operation when he had been so ill but they did not believe that he could help their son.

Now, at the end of his tether, John Tullett felt somehow Cain might be able to help.

To this day, he does not understand why he took this action.

Half-way through dialling, she found she could not do it and Lizette agreed to make the call, without hesitation. John Tullett thinks this incident was a pointer to the fact that it was destined that Lizette should be the one to make contact with John Cain, especially as she turned out to be so receptive.

Lizette returned. Cain had asked her where they all were and about Jason's condition and what relation she was to the boy. Cain instructed her to lay her hands on Jason's head. She never questioned these instructions but just carried them out.

John Tullett will never forget the occasion:

"Lizette placed her hands on Jason's head and almost immediately you could see by his face that the pain had subsided; his breathing became normal. It just happened too quickly for it to be coincidence. Then I noted that Lizette had slumped sideways and I had to support her.

"Her eyes were closed. A nurse had been taking Jason's temperature every half hour and now it registered nearly normal. Lizette recovered slightly and felt she had to leave the ward for a moment.

"Jason's pains suddenly returned and my wife and I tried separately to lay our hands on his head but it had no effect."

There followed an event which still astonishes John Tullett though he has related it to many reporters.

"Jason said repeatedly, 'No, I want Lizette. She knows how to do it'. Of course, I rushed to get her and as soon as she put her hands on the pains went again. Jason settled down and we were able to leave him and return home."

Lizette described later that she had felt heat and energy draining from her body through her hands and out into Jason's head. The next day she was utterly exhausted. Despite the heat she felt from her hands, Jason remarked that they had felt cool and soothing.

Jason slept well that night, experiencing no more acute pain but just discomfort from his scar.

Oddly enough, Lizette had not been at all frightened by her experiences and rang Cain to describe what had happened.

Cain suggested that John and Lizette should attend his public session the next afternoon to be "conditioned" so that they could assist in Jason's healing.

Several interesting phenomena occurred at this session.

Lizette went 'out' very quickly and concentrated on the double vision of which Jason had complained earlier at the hospital; he had only been able to see clearly by screwing up one eye. John Cain remarked that whilst she was in the altered state she must have been taking on Jason's eye condition, because she screwed up her eyes and could only open one eye when she 'came to'.

John Tullett experienced very little, he thought, except that when he stood up he felt as if there was a cushion of air beneath his feet and he wobbled. Cain said that he had been in an altered state.

John Tullett made a note of the time; it was 4.40 p.m. He had decided that from the first 'happening' in the hospital they would keep strict notes of times because he now believed anything might happen.

Lizette and he went straight over to the hospital.

To their amazement they found Jason's vision was perfectly normal. More astonishing was the fact that at exactly 4.40 p.m. (Sandy had also been watching the clock and Jason carefully), Jason had said, "Hello, dad," and had "seen" him at the foot of the bed.

Jason made steady progress from now on, with the occasional set-backs. He had discomfort as his scar knitted and once, severe constipation, both of which conditions Lizette "picked up" during a healing session, miles away in Bromborough!

Ten days after the operation Jason was allowed home, four or five days earlier than the hospital expected.

The evening of his homecoming, John Tullett asked his father-in-law, FRED SWARBRICK, of Victoria Road, Tranmere, to visit the healing session at Bromborough Civic Hall.

John Cain had said it would be beneficial to Jason if more of his family were there to concentrate on Jason's healing.

Fred was to discover, however, that the trip was to be of great benefit to himself!

When someone suggested that he should lie down on a mattress and have healing for a very painful back condition which had been the result of an accident at work seventeen years earlier, he said, "what's the use, I've been ill too long."

In addition to the back trouble, Fred had defective kidneys also caused by the accident.

He agreed, after persuasion by his family, to lie down and described afterwards terrific heat 'like an electric fire going right through my middle.'

When he climbed into John Tullett's car at the end of the evening, he did so without any trouble at all and later felt compelled to touch his toes.

He felt marvellous!

He had received an outright healing not only to his back but also to his kidneys.

A nice sequel to Fred's story is that his kidneys have been passed as Al for donation, which his doctor had said previously he could never hope to do.

To return to Jason's story:

He was taken regularly to John Cain for healing and both his father and Lizette, who was proving very receptive indeed and would often go 'out' if John Cain just walked into the room, were able to relieve Jason's headaches, which he still had.

John Tullett tells of how he would get up in the morning, go to Jason and together they would concentrate on Cains's photograph and John would put his hands on his son's head until the pain subsided.

By December, 1977, the hospital pronounced that if in eighteen months the symptoms had not recurred, then Jason was 'over the hill.'

Jason underwent a course of radio-therapy, followed by chemo-therapy, administered to reduce the size of the growth, although the hospital never committed themselves as to whether it would disappear altogether.

Cain continued to give the boy healing and although he tired easily, was underweight and could not attend school, he was practically symptom-free.

On June 3rd, 1978, John Tullett took Jason to a fun-fair but had to bring him home because of terrible headaches and sickness; the awful symptoms Jason had at the outset of his illness.

Cain had to give him a very long healing session before there was any relief.

This was obviously turning out to be a crucial stage in Jason's recovery, because ten days later, during a healing session at Bromborough, Jason became very distressed with his symptoms again. Cain spent nearly all evening with him and later accompanied him home and settled him to sleep.

Cain told the very worried parents that he considered that 'dispersal' was taking place. Their confidence in Cain was so strong they accepted his assessment without argument.

Unbeknown to the parents, Cain had told Fred Swarbrick around this time that the growth had gone.

On August 14th, the results of a scan done on July 19th – John Tullett recalls how dreadful that wait was – revealed that there was absolutely no trace of any growth!

The medical reaction was one of great surprise.

By September 21st, 1978, Jason returned to school and now leads a normal life.

It is important to state here that there was hospital treatment which may or may not have contributed to the disappearance of the growth, but John Tullett, previously a confirmed sceptic, has come

110

to some of his own conclusions:

"I have to acknowledge that John Cain has contributed a great deal to Jason's healing; it's something I can't be exact about but there is no denying that from that first 'phone call to him, many strange and inexplicable things have taken place."

Lizette and John have become helpers though pressure of work prevents John from devoting as much time as he would like. However, he sells John Cain's first book wherever he goes and mentions him every day.

"My whole outlook on life has been changed through meeting John Cain. I now enjoy helping others more and I realise how much more important it is to have health and emotional happiness. I am also closer to my son than ever before and make time to play with him.

"The contact we have as a family with John Cain is very important psychologically to all of us."

# VI

As stated earlier, of all aspects of Cain's healing methods, Absent Healing is the one most difficult to comprehend and explain.

And yet there are letters by the score in Cain's files from grateful patients from all over the country.

Each of the ones I read, told a different story about suffering relieved, of hope renewed, of sometimes, even, a complete cure!

All of them were from people who had never set eyes on Cain unless they had seen his photograph in a newspaper article.

MRS JUNE WAKELAM aged 41 from 83 Crescent Drive, Ellesmere Port, Merseyside, slipped a disc in 1976. She should have stayed in bed, on a board, but with a young family and a husband on shift-work, it was impossible.

She was out shopping one day and called in at her mother-in-law's at the same time as a relation who was receiving treatment from Cain. He suggested that he should telephone Cain and make an appointment for her.

Cain said he would link-up with her there and then and instructed June's relation to hold his photograph against her spine. June reports that she felt vibrations immediately in her spine and within minutes the 'agonising' pain had eased. She was able to stand and sit without any pain whatsoever.

She was utterly amazed by what happened and has had no recurrence of her back trouble since!

\* \* \* \* \*

It is surprising how often the phrase "pull yourself together" is used by psychiatrists. When it was said to MRS IRENE ANDREW, of Westminster Road, Macclesfield, she had been suffering from agoraphobia for eighteen years!

The fears she had about going out on her own were so real that she became totally dependent on someone accompanying her. Since she had not been told *how* to 'pull herself together' she felt totally alone with her problem.

She wrote to John Cain after reading about him in an article. She reports that when she received a reply from him on May 28th 1979, her healing began almost immediately. Most noticeable was the lack of tension; there was no more perspiring at the thought of going anywhere by herself. Gradually, she found she could catch the bus, visit friends and shop by herself. To most of us this might not sound much of an achievement, but, in Irene's words, 'it was like being released from prison'.

This wonderful healing came about just through reading John Cain's comforting letter, compiled by his wife, Audrey.

*     *     *     *     *

Sometimes a patient can receive Absent Healing when a member of the family contacts John Cain unbeknown to the patient.

This happened to THOMAS ZUGER, aged 25 from Bromborough, Merseyside.

His mother had received Absent Healing herself unbeknownst to her when a friend asked Cain to heal her eczema. He did and only when her friend told her that she had been put on Cain's Absent Healing list, did Thomas' mother know why her hands had suddenly healed!

Thomas developed eczema on his legs in 1977 and had been using a cortisone-based ointment for months with no success. His mother asked Cain to put Thomas on his Absent Healing list but never told her son what she had done.

One day, she asked him casually if his condition was better. To her surprise he said that it was quite better. Then she told him that he had been receiving Absent Healing from Cain!

MISS LORNA BARLOW of Grange Road, Layton, Blackpool, was at her brother's house when she read the *NEWS OF THE WORLD article* about Cain. Not a paper she usually bought, she was impressed enough with the article to send off a letter to one of Cain's patients whose address was printed in the newspaper. She asked him to pass on her letter to Cain. She had no idea when her letter would be received by Cain but whilst she was waiting for a reply she reports that one morning, she woke with what she can only describe as 'upliftment' of her spirit and complete disappearance of the 'agonising' pain in her right arm. She had been unable to use her arm for fifteen months.

She just did not know what had happened to her and thought in fact a 'miracle' had taken place. Also, she felt great relief from the pain from curvature of the spine.

Two or three days later, she received Cain's printed letter stating that from the moment he had received her letter, 'the healing intercession had commenced'.

Lorna then knew that she had indeed received instant healing from Cain before she had even heard from him!

\*     \*     \*     \*     \*

MRS LUCY WARING, aged 58 from Blackburn, Lancashire, also began to feel better as soon as she had written off to John Cain in May, 1979. She noticed that the pain and heartburn resulting from a chronic duodenal ulcer condition, diagnosed in December, 1978, had both subsided. Gradually she reports that she began to feel better all round. Continuing the link-up with Cain most evenings, she says that she always benefits greatly from the relaxation she receives when looking at his photograph and 'tuning-in' with him. Sometimes, she says she feels intense heat also.

She can now carry shopping bags, take her very energetic dog for walks and not cringe with pain when he pulls her!

She takes no medicines but is just sensible about diet.

# VII

THE REV. BILL STRIBLEY, Minister of the West Kirby Unitarian Free Christian Church, Wirral, and joint minister of the Matthew Henry Chapel, Blacon, Chester, testified to the genuineness of John Cain as a healer in Cain's first book "Heal, My Son!".

He has never ceased to admire Cain and has this to say about him:

"I've attended many of John Cain's sessions," he says, "and I must say from the outset, that I'm not easily swayed: I'm both a Doctor of Philosophy and a Psychologist.

I feel there's only one answer to Cain's healing gift. He is being used as a channel and people like him will always find it hard to be believed.

"But I'll always stand by him and think, if anything, that over the years his gift grows stronger. I have seen acquaintances of mine healed by him and they have maintained their 'cure'.

"People expect a Minister of a church to be criticised for standing up and speaking in favour of Cain, but I've actually had letters congratulating me for taking such a stand."

# VIII

John Cain always maintains that he does not need the back-up of scientists, doctors or theologians to convince him that his work is genuine: "I'm just interested in making people better," he always says.

But an increasing number of experts are expressing interest in John Cain's work.

\* \* \* \* \*

NORMAN CRAINE, a chemist from Cheshire, was introduced to the work of Cain by the Reverend Bill Stribley who has himself followed the healing of Cain with great interest for a number of years.

Mr. Craine decided to attend a public demonstration Cain was to give at the Philharmonic Hall, Liverpool, in September, 1977.

Craine saw the opening of the session which always follows the same procedure at such meetings.

To elucidate:

Cain usually stands alone on the platform. Some visitors have already been seated on mattresses, others on chairs.

The music which is played during the first few minutes John Cain is on the stage and which probably helps to focus the audience's attention, is quite loud at this point, but fades slowly into the background as the session proceeds.

It is strange to see for the first time people fall back on to the mattresses or just slump their heads forward if they are sitting in chairs. Cain describes this moment as 'the fusion of minds'. They appear to enter an 'altered state of consciousness' and Cain further explains that at this moment their personal healing begins.

Norman Craine recalls that seated in the audience at the Philharmonic Hall, he did not seem to be affected in any way during the 'fusion of minds' but he saw many extraordinary things and came away fascinated.

It was only the next day when he discovered that a stiff neck which had troubled him for two years had become 'free' did he wonder whether he had benefited from any healing!

A qualified pharmacist with over thirty years' experience, running his own business and coming into frequent contact with members of the medical profession, with many of whom he is on very friendly terms, he might be thought to be more than usually sceptical of the authenticity of healing.

Craine says:

"I have acquired considerable knowledge of orthodox medical treatment. Whilst being fully aware of the bad publicity given in the press to many drugs (some of it, I admit, justifiable), I also know that without them millions of lives would have been lost.

"My father, who died, aged 77 in 1960, would almost certainly have died twenty years earlier from pernicious anaemia but for the discovery of Vitamin B12. My mother would no doubt have had a much shorter life except for penicillin which cured her of double pneumonia. And my brother owes his existence to the fact he was cured of T.B. by the then new practice of chemotherapy.

"I want to make it quite clear that my interest in healing is not due to disillusionment with orthodox treatment.

"It must, however, be admitted that drugs are imperfect instruments of healing.

"For example, an aspirin, taken for a headache, does not confine its activity to the head. It is absorbed into the blood stream, affecting all parts of the body, sometimes producing unpleasant side-effects."

From the first time Norman Craine visited one of John Cain's group healing sessions, he openly admits that his life has taken on a new dimension.

"On the first visit," he says, "I took an arthritic friend with me who had tried every known antiflammatory drug without much relief and suffered gastritis as a result. The improvement in his condition after one session was phenomenal.

"Though comparatively healthy myself, I had been troubled for years with migraine-type headaches and a painful back due to a lumbar injury.

"Since my first treatment I have been almost completely free from both these complaints."

Mr. Craine took along another friend who, after weeks of varied treatment by his doctor for a severe case of haemorrhoids, was now incapacitated by this condition. He went twice, was completely 'cured' and has had no trouble since.

Craine feels he should clarify what the word 'cure' means to him:

"I can only say that the patients I have seen at John Cain's, in addition to my personal friends, have become symptom-free, and have stayed that way.

"I have been tremendously impressed.

"I am aware that healing is open to abuse by charlatans and by misguided people who imagine they possess gifts which in fact militate against the good name of healing. But it is not logical to suppose that natural healing does not exist.

"I have always felt instinctively there was some universal force capable of putting things in good order."

Norman Craine has been observing Cain for many months now and acknowledges him along with many others as one of the great healers of our time.

"John Cain is coping mainly with people who have found orthodox medicine not entirely helpful and with those who have simply lost hope. Thus the odds are very heavily against him because many come to him with no faith, indeed probably most are sceptics.

"But I can honestly say that I have not met anyone who hasn't received benefit of some kind, whether it be physical or spiritual.

"Some time ago Cain invited me to become one of his helpers and I have been acutely aware of the healing power he is able to channel in this way. Working with him has given me great joy and satisfaction, and I am absolutely convinced that Cain possesses a truly remarkable gift and believe that anyone who knows of his work and fails to acknowledge this is being less than honest.

"If I may be permitted a dream, it is that the medical profession and people like John Cain will one day work together in harmony, each complementing the other.

"When that day comes I'm sure a tremendous step forward will have been made in the practice of healing".

\*   \*   \*   \*   \*

# IX

RON BAKER, one-time General Secretary of The Spiritualists' National Union Limited, calls John Cain a "truly modern healer, bringing forward ancient methods into the modern world. He heals the four-fold personality: the physical, the emotional, mental and spiritual."

Mr. Baker has been interested in healing for thirty years and has witnessed an interesting selection of healing methods. He finds Cain difficult to fit into the more usual categories of the healing field.

"John Cain," Mr. Baker believes, "evokes strong feelings; people are either strongly attracted or repelled by his type of personality. But there is no doubt at all that he has charisma, not in a pretentious way because he will often go out of his way to present an image of 'I don't care a damn'! He's truly an individual not needing or relying on other experts in the field. He has had more than a fair share of criticism from within spiritualist circles where jealousy and envy are often rife. But he just carries on healing and leaves the experts floundering in the quagmire of their theories.

"He does not consciously assert personal ideas into his healing but simply allows healing to take place through him. I cannot think of anyone else in my years of experience who has opened up this method of healing other than John Cain."

Mr. Baker firmly believes that the whole spiritual experience pivots on the 'altered state of consciousness' and whereas many healers go into trance to heal, with Cain the opposite is true and it is the patient whose state is altered.

"For years," he says, "I've used my own gifts to pass on messages from the higher world to those in this world; I can only remember one person going into a trance whilst I was talking, but with Cain it happens continually. A rich field of exploration and research could be opened up. Through this contact, the spiritual aspect of a person is touched upon; not just the religious aspect because John Cain is universal and people's barriers are cut across.

"The physical manipulations which occur during healing sessions without any contact with Cain are, as far as I know, quite unique.

119

The only comparison I can possibly think of are the ecstatic states which primitive peoples are capable of attaining due to their closeness to nature.

"John Cain is connected with the natural element of things and projects a strong magnetic field which because of its strength needs no expert to discern. The gift must continue unspoiled so that it will evolve in the future.

"Many people have cause to be grateful, including myself, for the help John Cain has given them. And I am pleased to say John Cain is a friend of mine."

# X

DR DONALD BLYTHING is a lecturer in psychology and has a private practice as a consultant psychologist on Merseyside.

He specialises in careers guidance and in specific learning problems of children and adults.

"I first heard of John Cain," he says, "when he healed the fiancée of a relation of mine. She had become suddenly blind and after only one visit to Cain, her sight returned slightly, and after three visits it had returned completely.

"She had been told it was a neurological blindness and had been to many doctors and specialists but with no success. I had been so impressed by this healing, that I went along to see Cain at work.

"I considered him to be a genuine and sincere person doing dedicated work."

Dr Blything, on that first visit to observe Cain, allowed himself to be put into a relaxed state.

"I felt very relaxed and a headache that had been troublesome was lifted during the healing session I received."

Dr Blything feels that more people in the caring professions should consider John Cain's work with an open mind.

"He is doing very worth-while work and this should not be underestimated.

"In my work, I have come to realise that if people are to get better, they have to want to be cured; they have got to get out of rigid behaviour and thinking patterns. From my observations of John Cain, I believe he can help people to do this."

Dr Blything has spoken to many people who have received benefit from Cain for depression and anxiety states resulting from living alone, fears and doubts about life and death and bereavement.

He says:

"Cain helped another relation of mine who was in a very low state for some time after bereavement. Cain calmed her and she is now able to cope with her loss much better."

Donald acknowledges that Cain can complement his own work because in treating a case of adult learning disability, for example, it

121

is most important for the adult to learn to relax and be calm before his problem can be coped with.

"I have often told such a client," Dr Blything says, "that seeing Cain could open the mind and help in coming to terms with the problem. Where a client has taken my advice it has indeed proved very beneficial.

"I've observed the people who visit John Cain and it is my view that the majority of them have either become disillusioned with the medical profession or that orthodox medical treatment can no longer help them. To them John Cain is the last resort and he is giving them a glimmer of light. In some cases, he has had remarkable results.

"It is not easy to say what takes place during a healing session. All I can say is that I can induce an altered state of consciousness with the use of hypnotherapy. But I acknowledge that John Cain has superior gifts in this field and would say that his ability to induce the altered state 'en masse' is extraordinary and extremely beneficial."

# XI

MALCOLM HUGHES, M.Sc., B. Sc., is a lecturer at Birmingham Polytechnic in the Department of Bio-medical Science.

His association with John Cain came about through his specialist knowledge of bio-medicine and, in particular, the area of research in which he works, namely, psychosomatic medicine.

"It has long been acknowledged," Mr Hughes says, "that the human mind possesses capabilities far more extensive than many give credit for. The mind in the form of conscious and subconscious actions can, when under stress precipitate a wide variety of physical symptoms and disorders relating to all body systems. Under such conditions, conventional drug treatment, while able to alleviate discomfort, may often fail to cure the condition completely.

"To bring about complete recovery from psychosomatic-type conditions, it is becoming evident that treatment of the source of the condition, i.e. the subject's mind (or emotional state) is required. An acceptable level of success has been obtained by myself and others by the use of psychotherapeutic means, often with the use of hypnosis."

Because of his experience in this area of treatment, Malcolm Hughes was requested by a publisher, who was interested in John Cain's work, to observe at close quarters a demonstration to be given by Cain in the presence of a large audience, together with the press, at the Liverpool Philharmonic Hall in September, 1977.

Mr Hughes says:

"My purpose was to act as an objective observer, and afterwards, to report to a publisher on what conclusions I had arrived at concerning Cain's approach and method of treatment.

"While having familiarised myself with the subject of faith healing, it became immediately apparent that Cain's approach took on a different aspect to that more often encountered. My main concern was not only how treatment was administered, but also the effect, both physically and psychologically upon the subjects undergoing treatment.

"Within the Hall there was no shortage of patients of both sexes and covering virtually the entire age spectrum. A vast number

123

showed signs of various musculo-skeletal disorders, which include arthritis, osteo-arthritis, rheumatism, displacement of vertebral discs, frozen shoulder, sciatica."

Mr Hughes accompanied Cain in his examination of each subject in the Hall that night and observed that the majority exhibited moderate to severe forms of their conditions.

"I noticed that all had been 'induced' into a comatose position and appeared to vary in their degrees of consciousness. First impressions ruled out the use of hypnotic techniques in the inducement of this state. This was further substantiated by some of the subjects later, as the state they described as entering into bore little resemblance to that experienced by subjects undergoing hypnosis.

"The extent to which suggestion of any form was applied was also questionable. Among the twenty or so subjects treated and closely observed by me was a child of not more than three years of age. To my mind, such a subject would be too young to be aware of the severity of her condition, let alone to have built up a faith that a person such as John Cain would have the ability to cure her. Yet, as with the other subjects, including a handful of sceptics, she too adopted an 'altered state' for the duration of the session."

Having borne witness to the events that occurred on that evening, as well as considering evidence provided by other subjects, Mr Hughes acknowledges that these people with a variety of disorders, notably of the musculo-skeletal type, underwent a remarkable and in terms of orthodox medicine, an unexplained cure.

He makes these final points:

'No obvious reason for these results is apparent. The extent to which paranormal factors enter the situation remain a possibility, for despite advances in the technology used, there are limitations in determining what forces may be manifest in the treatment afforded by Cain. Certainly, in his own way, he apparently succeeds where conventional medicine sadly seems to fail".

# XII

Before and during the writing of this book I made enquiries at healing centres and sanctuaries throughout the country. I believe I carried out these journalistic investigations without bias and objectively.

I soon discovered that there are hundreds of healers, many of them working part-time only, who feel that they can help people in need. Very few of them demand exorbitant charges for their services; they rely – as does John Cain – on voluntary donations.

More disturbing was my discovery of so-called clinics where professional 'healers' practise. Often they call themselves 'spiritual hypnotherapist' or some such fanciful names. Their fees are very steep indeed: one of them asks for £10. – consulting fee for the first brief session and £100.– for a further four sessions to follow. He claims to cure disorders, such as depression, insomnia and lack of confidence, all of which I have seen cured by John Cain 'free of charge'.

Another centre charges £5.– for a half-hour session, explaining that they have to meet expenses. However, they assured me also that they would not turn back somebody who could not pay five pounds.

'Psychic surgeons' ask for anything between £10.– and £100.–, and the money is always referred to as a voluntary donation; but several journalists have written about guidance which is given to voluntary donors and the psychological pressure which is exercised to make those donations conform to the expectations of the 'healers'.

I also concluded very soon that one is expected to pay according to the performance; BBC television has shown some superb demonstrations of method acting, and some of those healers would do well in hospital soap operas.

John Cain is a full-time healer; but in all those months I have investigated and explored his activities, there has never been a mention about money or fees. Hundreds come every week to his healing sessions; most of them leave a donation in a little envelope or on a table at the back of the hall, but I have also seen quite a number who could obviously ill afford to leave anything, who left quietly

125

without making a donation. Yet I never saw anybody follow them and ask for money. But I did see, on more than one occasion, John Cain quietly slipping a note into the palm of an old age pensioner who had come for healing.

Cain works seven days a week; if he is not engaged in personal or contact healing, he is on the telephone, which, as I mentioned earlier, never seems to stop ringing at 20 North Road in Birkenhead. He occasionally visits his patients at home when they are too ill to come to him or he goes into hospitals, often to be with a patient in his last hours, but unfortunately he cannot make as many house visits as he would like to make because of his healing commitments at the centre.

I became saddened and sometimes frustrated when I observed, whilst writing this book, how stubborn, even bloody-minded some of the medical authorities were. One 'spokesman' of the British Medical Association actually said: "John Cain? – If he is one of those faith healers, we have never heard of him. We know nothing about that kind and type of healing."

What utter nonsense! I know for a fact that the 'spokesman' had heard of John Cain and so had many members of the Association. For weeks the newspapers had been full of stories about John Cain, and most articles carried quotes from B.M.A. spokesmen; even if they had not heard about him in the beginning, they certainly must have been curious why so many journalists enquired about that 'healer'.

What are they afraid of? I have asked myself many times why the medical authorities don't investigate such healing phenomena as we journalists do. They could at least find out what it is all about and stop making a laughing stock of themselves by repeating total ignorance of the existence of healing.

We cannot live without our doctors, surgeons, nurses and many essential medicines and drugs. I was brought up on penicillin and antibiotics. I experienced major surgery and, indeed, I would not be here to write this book without the dedicated and selfless devotion of doctors, surgeons and nurses. I would have died when I was twelve years old without the help of surgeons. Nothing is further from my mind than to attack or 'knock' the medical profession.

But as a journalist I must always balance one fact against another, one allegation against another allegation and one statement against another statement. I was deeply dismayed when I encountered such apathy and total disinterest from the spokesmen of national medical associations. Thankfully, this apathy is not shared by all doctors and surgeons. I have seen some learned, medical men at Cain's healing demonstrations. They come as private individuals, and when it becomes known that they are doctors or surgeons, they ask for their privacy to be respected.

I have no cause to go back on my promise I made each and every time. I have spoken to several eminent medical men, who do not share the ignorance or arrogance of the official spokesmen. On the contrary, I always cherish the enthusiasm and encouragement given to John Cain – and to me, his biographer in a lesser way – by these doctors who had come to see for themselves. I have refrained from using their names in this book, nor have I found it necessary to tell John Cain's story with anonymous comments. Those who have testified to healing, knew that I was going to write about their experiences for a newspaper or in a book; they all gave me permission, not only to tell their stories but to give their names and addresses as well. They were all prepared to stand up and be counted.

Some patients who have come to John Cain for help and whom I interviewed begged me not to give their names because they feared – with good cause, I am sorry to say – that their doctors would refuse to give them any further treatment if they were to see a healer. John Cain always feels very sad for those whom he knows he could help but who are prevented from seeking it for such reasons.

Only recently pain research clinics have been opened throughout the country; one such clinic, specialising in the investigation of back troubles is under consideration for Merseyside. From my observations, it appears that Cain has outstanding success in these two areas particularly. Surely, this would be an ideal opportunity of looking at the extraordinary gifts of John Cain, and some other healers, and to ascertain whether their 'secret' of diminishing pain and often vanquishing it, is really so secret!

How else can I finish my task but by dedicating this book to all those hundreds of people whom I have interviewed, to the thousands who have gone to John Cain for healing and received it, and to the thousands who are yet to go to him.

They all have been and will be feeling much the better for it, not only physically, but spiritually also. Life and health to them will indeed seem a precious possession.

## PUBLISHER'S NOTE

Following the publication of *HEAL, MY SON!*, many readers of the book telephoned the publishers for an appointment with Mr. John Cain. Of course, we are in no position to assist readers in this respect and we have therefore taken the precaution to obtain such information as may help those who want to get in touch with the Healer himself:

John Cain restricts his healing practice to Merseyside. Anyone who wishes to obtain information about healing centres, dates and time, is advised to write to:

John Cain
20 North Road,
Birkenhead,
Merseyside.

Mr. Cain has no objection if in cases of urgency and emergency people telephone him (051) 652 5089, but he advises patients strongly against calling at 20 North Road, Birkenhead, without a prior appointment because he does not want to disappoint callers.

The publishers hope that the above information will be useful and they suggest that all enquiries should be made directly to Mr. John Cain and not to them.